SEXUALLY SATISFIED COUPLE

Sex Makes Relationship Sweeter "Best Sex Satisfaction Guide Book for Singles Dating To Be Married and Married Couples" Ignite Your Sexual Dreams

By

HARDY SHARON KHALIFA

TABLE OF CONTENT

CHAPTER ONE
INTRODUCTION

So you want to know how to make your woman feel good in bed. First of all, well done. You're prepared to put in the time and effort necessary to make sure she finds new heights of pleasure in her private moments with you, in a world where far too many men are too preoccupied with their own pleasure to be concerned about their partners'. You want to express to your woman how much she means to you, obviously. No better way to make her feel special than to indulge her erotic cravings?

Satisfying a woman sexually can bring immense joy and positive vibes for your relationships, as strong chemistry between you and her can result in increased closeness and intimacy. It can be difficult to understand the subtleties of female pleasure because women usually take longer than men to feel sexually aroused. But this mystery is easily solved if you truly try to figure out what your partner's sexual preferences are. In addition, your woman will be ready to roar once you kindle the fire of arousal, and you might be caught off guard by her raw side. That is unquestionably worth the entire effort.

There are techniques to increase her pleasure in sex if you want her to want you even more. Tricks, erogenous zones, and postures that will make her twitch her toes and arch her back in lustful delight. You don't have to spend your time learning the specifics of female pleasure on your own. To help you figure out how to make your girl feel good in bed, we are here. Let's look at the parts of her body that require attention so that she consistently

receives an O.

SEXUAL SATISFACTION

The desire for and enjoyment of sex by women has

historically received little attention. Women's access to

sexual activities was severely restricted for centuries in

the Western world; as a result, they were forced to visit

their doctor for "treatment" (genital massages) in order to

alleviate their sexual frustration. Thankfully, the idea that

women can have and enjoy sex just as much as men does,

and that everyone has the right to a satisfying sexual

relationship, has gradually gained traction. The definition

of sexual satisfaction and how to achieve it have come

under closer scrutiny in research as a result of this

paradigm change.

WHAT REALLY IS SEXUAL SATISFACTION?

Lawrance and Byers, well-known figures in the field of sexual satisfaction, have defined sexual satisfaction as "an effective response arising from one's subjective evaluation of the positive and negative dimensions associated with one's sexual relationship", which is one of the most well-liked and frequently used definitions of the term. To put it another way, sexual satisfaction is the feeling you get from your sexual life when you weigh its pros and cons.

Depending on the aspects of sexuality that are most significant to each individual, people's perceptions of what constitutes sexual satisfaction in public may differ. In general, though, having positive feelings about your sexuality—like pleasure and desire—as well as your sexual relationship—like a sense of intimacy and bonding with your partner—are necessary for you to be content with your sexual life.

IS SEXUAL SATISFACTION EVEN THAT IMPORTANT?

Not only does sexual satisfaction affect your sexual well-being, but it also has a significant impact on your personal and interpersonal health. More specifically: Higher quality of life, as well as better general health and wellbeing, are reported by sexually satisfied people than by those who are not. Sensual satisfaction in the bedroom is associated with improved mental health, including reduced symptoms of anxiety and depression, especially for new moms. Thus, make sure to utilize the baby's naps to the fullest. Sexual fulfillment and the quality of relationships are closely correlated for both men and women. It is true that people who are happier in their sexual lives are also happier in their relationships, are more devoted to them, and feel more love for their partners.

A higher level of sexual wellbeing is also correlated with sexual satisfaction. People who are satisfied sexually tend to report higher levels of desire, arousal, and regular orgasms. Sexual satisfaction is not always predicted by sexual functioning, which includes experiencing desire, becoming aroused and "wet," having an orgasm, and not experiencing pain. The good news is that you can still feel sexually satisfied in spite of having sexual issues!

WHAT FACTORS AFFECT SEXUAL SATISFACTION?

Numerous aspects of your life are correlated with sexual satisfaction. The following factors could influence one's level of sexual satisfaction:

Increased sexual satisfaction:

- Having an internalized homophobia or low sexual guilt

- Posing with confidence and assertiveness

- Sexting more frequently

- Taking part in a wider range of sexual activities

- Having social support and a good partner

- Cohabiting with a spouse

- Being in a committed relationship or married

- Enjoying and being more intimate in relationships

Decreased level of sexual satisfaction

- Experiencing sexual distress, (which is defined as worrying, frustrated, or anxious about one's sexual life)

- Exhibiting signs of anxiety and depression

- Feeling pressured

- Experiencing problems with sex (erectile dysfunction, dry vagina, pain during sex)

- Adultery

HOW CAN SEXUAL SATISFACTION INCREASE?

The quick response is to talk and cuddle. Though research has shown that people in both dating and long-term relationships who talk to their partner about their sexual likes and dislikes report greater sexual satisfaction, communication may be easier said than done. Thus, don't be scared to let your partner know where you enjoy and dislike receiving kisses.

An additional factor in your sexual satisfaction may be your post-sex routine. People who hug, kiss, and converse deeply after sex report feeling more satisfied with their romantic and sexual relationships, according to recent research. Therefore, give yourself some time before getting out of bed (or the couch, or the floor, or

wherever you ended up).

CHAPTER TWO

A SEXLESS MARRIAGE: WHAT IS IT?

A marriage that lacks intimacy between the partners is referred to as a sexless marriage. Experts state that any marriage with ten or fewer sexual activity sessions in a year can be classified as sexless since different couples have different sexual expectations and desires. This depends on the couple, though, as some can still have healthy relationship sex once a week or once a month. You can declare that you are in a sexless marriage if, during the last few months, your sexual life has either drastically decreased or vanished entirely.

An investigation conducted in 2019 found that 19% of 659 couples were in what is known as a "sexless marriage." The majority of couples in this group reported having only had one or two intimate encounters in the previous year, and some of them said they hadn't had any kind of sexual contact in over a year. By contrast, approximately 35% of the married couples reported having sex one to three times a month, 25% said they enjoyed sex every week, and 21% said they enjoyed sex a few times a week, which is a healthy amount of sex life.

They say that marriages are made in heaven, but we still have to work at keeping them together. Most couples tend to overlook the subtle but significant differences between living together and staying together. You don't truly "live" together and truly get to know someone until you are married. For this reason, some couples who have been dating for a very short time have a strong marriage, while there are cases where couples who have been together for well over ten years separate after getting married.

Joining two cultures, people, families, values, customs, and a host of other intangibles together is the essence of marriages. Knowing each other well enough to communicate without becoming overly attached is one of the things you need to know in order to keep your marriage intact. Though at first it might seem like a difficult undertaking, as you develop as a person and in your marriage, you begin to notice the small cracks where you might want to apply adhesive or apply a bandage, and that is how you learn. In this fast-paced world where divorces are more common than solutions, surviving and maintaining a marriage is especially important. To start, focus on what you can control.

Are you starting to notice that you and your spouse aren't getting enough sex? Are the sex experiences traumatizing? You're not making the ascent when you would like to? Does giving always mean receiving nothing in return? Do you often want to be physically intimate with your partner but your partner rejects your requests? You might be stuck in a rut if you answered "yes" to any of these questions. Lack of sex can destroy your marriage in the same way that emotional lack of availability or distancing can. Its effects are more pervasive and have the potential to grow into a bigger issue by leaking into other marital cracks. Lack of sex in a marriage or having no sex at all can cause serious problems.

REASONS FOR A
SEXLESS MARRIAGE

The frequency of sex in a marriage can fluctuate for a number of reasons. Mismatched libidos are a common problem in marriages, which strains the individual with a higher libido when their partner is unable to fulfill their sexual needs. A lack of sex in a marriage can be caused by a variety of factors, although mismatched libido is the most common cause.

Among the most frequent reasons are:

A MEDICAL CONDITION OR HEALTH ISSUE: The level of intimacy and sex drive in your spouse may conscious about their appearance—is one of the most frequent causes of sexless marriages. They voluntarily reject the experience of intimacy, which becomes routine. It gets harder and harder to handle over time, and you start to wonder what went wrong.

EFFECTS OF LACK OF SEX IN MARRIAGE

If both partners feel satisfied with a marriage that does not include sex, it may not be a problem for that relationship. They may find other ways to show intimacy, such as kissing, cuddling, or spending time together. In some cases, one or both partners might identify as asexual, a sexual orientation defined by a lack of sexual attraction. In these cases, it may be normal for a be influenced by their general physical or mental health. Health problems also interfere with regular physiological functions, such as arousal in certain individuals. Your spouse's decreased sex drive could be the result of a recent health issue.

MENOPAUSE: There is a strong correlation between menopause and sexless marriages, as the former influences hormonal levels and the latter is one of the main causes of sexless marriages. It's important to keep in mind that even though sex may not be discussed during these times, partners should still show each other affection in other ways to ensure that they feel valued and wanted.

INJURY/TRAUMA: It may have long-lasting effects on your married sex life if your spouse has unresolved sexual trauma experiences from her past. Sexual trauma alters the brain's association between physical intimacy and feelings of fear, manipulation, force, and shame, which has an impact on the body's reaction to intimacy.

DEPRESSION: Depression is another factor in sexless marriages. Relationships suffer when an individual becomes disinterested in life and experiences hopelessness or restlessness. It's important to get help when you or your partner experience mental health issues. In this instance, having no sex in a marriage should be the least of your worries because these circumstances could have disastrous effects if you don't get professional assistance.

CHILDBIRTH: Although most medical professionals recommend waiting four to six weeks after giving birth, the American College of Obstetricians and Gynecologists (ACOG) states that there is no set period of time after childbirth when women are ready for sex. A woman's body may not always feel ready for intimacy right away. Additionally, most women find that having a newborn supersedes their need for physical intimacy.

LACK OF GOOD COMMUNICATION: It becomes challenging to keep up a healthy sexual relationship when you're dealing with a lot of relationship issues. Low sexual desire from your partner can be caused by a variety of factors, such as negative emotions, unresolved relationship issues, infidelity, addiction to masturbation, and passive-aggressive behavior.

Many people are misinformed about sex and the act of romantic relationships, which frequently results in the development of unhealthy relationships. For example, most people think that having sex should be unplanned, so most couples wait for it to happen naturally, but it never does.

INSUFFICIENT FOREPLAY: Without much or any foreplay, many partners jump right in. This is among the main causes of the other partner's disinterest. It takes longer for women to become excited and aroused for sex, which is why foreplay becomes crucial. Thus, enjoy every moment of your "alone time" by moving slowly, being inventive, and spending enough time in foreplay.

MUCH STRESS: An individual's sex drive is impacted by excessive stress, which also has an impact on their physical and mental health. The stress hormone cortisol is produced by the brain during times of stress, and it lowers libido. Furthermore, stress exacerbates feelings of exhaustion, anxiety, and frazzlement, which further exacerbates the desire for sex.

ADVERSE DRUG REACTIONS: The fact that many prescribed drugs have side effects that could impair their ability to have sexual relations surprises a lot of people. Let's say you find it uncomfortable or intolerable that your medication appears to be negatively affecting your sex drive. In that situation, it is best to speak with your doctor to find out if your suspicions are valid and to discuss any possible replacements that may be recommended.

IRRATIONAL SEXUAL ACTIONS: It has nothing to do with men or women. Someone who takes an absurdly high view of having fun with sex can be the biggest buzzkiller. Irrational sexual behaviors are unacceptable, even if they are the most personal choice. You can go see a sexologist if you and your partner are having trouble changing this behavior.

LOW SEX OR DIFFERENT DRIVES: It is uncommon for a couple's sex drives to mesh perfectly. No matter how sexually active a couple is, if they both lose their libido or don't value sex as much as their friendship, sense of emotional security, and other aspects of their marriage, it can still work out. Finding a delicate balance between meeting each other's needs and not pressuring them to have physical intimacy when they don't want to can be challenging for couples whose sexual drives are mismatched. However, that does not imply that a couple experiencing problems with their sex has gone too far. Actually, in order to salvage their relationship, they really need to be willing to have difficult talks and seek professional help from a therapist or sexologist.

UNRESOLVED DISPUTES: Although disagreements are inevitable in a relationship, if you allow them to fester, your bond will deteriorate. You feel isolated in a relationship when there are unresolved conflicts. Occasionally, one partner becomes distracted and, instead of fostering intimacy, allows disagreements to sabotage their sex life.

LACK OF CONCERN: Physical distance between people can be one of several indicators that a relationship is failing. You may already be over your partner if you can picture yourself waking up with someone else or by yourself.

There is nothing worse than ignoring or feeling embarrassed to talk about sexual problems when they arise. To keep a marriage intact, both partners need to be willing to talk things out before they become hostile to one another and file for divorce. Losing responsibility and caring for your spouse is one of the most underappreciated causes of a sexless marriage.

POOR PERSONAL HYGIENE: One crucial component that, if overlooked, can interfere with your intimacy rituals is hygiene. By keeping your personal areas clean, you can avoid embarrassing situations and infections, as well as improve your sexual health. A few things to keep in mind are: Wear clean underwear, keep your privates tidy, cut off your pubic hair, and avoid oral sex if you both have genital sores. You should think about seeing a specialist and supporting your partner confidently if they are afflicted with an infection.

INAPPROPRIATE MOTIVES FOR COHABITATION: While children are impacted by divorce, they may suffer greater harm from unhappy parents. Time does not change the fact that all you have in common are the kids and "date nights" or "together alone." That does not bode well. If you are with your partner for more than just romantic reasons, you may be compromising on a lot of things that you are still unaware of.

BODY MODIFICATIONS: Body change—when one or both partners gain weight or begin to feel self-

relationship not to have sex or to have a low amount of sex. For others, a lack of sex becomes a problem and can have a number of negative impacts on the relationship, including the following.

Affects Marital Self-Esteem: Your sense of self-worth and confidence can be damaged by not having sex. You may begin to feel as though something is wrong with you and that it is affecting other areas. You might become overly self-conscious, which could have a bad effect on other aspects of your life besides your relationship, such as your career. If a partner doesn't think they're sexually attractive or desirable, they might have low self-esteem. They might think their partner doesn't think they're attractive, or they might think there's a problem with their bodies. Sometimes they might think it's awkward for their partner to see them in their underwear or that they can't be vulnerable with them.

Random Thoughts Regarding Marriage: Despite the fact that this may seem like a very nebulous situation, the ongoing unhappiness can cause you to have a variety of confusing thoughts about your marriage and yourself.

Advice: It's best to hear it straight from the source to clear your mind of any confusion. Take a seat with your partner, be as open and honest as you can about your position, and let the dialogue guide you toward a resolution. Be cautious, sincere, and polite.

Misconceptions/misunderstandings: Misunderstandings are one of the major effects of not having sex in a marriage. When you and your partner are upset about something, the frustration can build and manifest itself in different ways. Now that sexual frustration erupts, it messes everything up even more!

Instability and Uncertainty: If you find it difficult to talk about sex, you may think that your relationship is about to end. You might observe a weakening of your emotional bond and an increasing sense of distance between you and your partner. The stability of the marriage may suffer if partners start to drift apart.

Absence of Closeness: Intimacy can take many different forms besides sexual relations, such as meaningful conversation, caressing, holding hands, and kissing. When there is less sex, partners may notice a decline in other forms of intimacy.

Advice: Take a deep breath, wait ten seconds before responding, and avoid getting into a fight or argument.

Sensations of Being Alone: Sexless marriages can occasionally end sooner than they otherwise would have. Feelings of loneliness brought on by low self-esteem may begin to surface. In general, emotional closeness and affection can suffer, sometimes to the point of separation or divorce.

Discontent: Couples who are unhappy in their marriage as a whole may yearn for more sex or feel unsatisfied with their current sexual life. They can struggle to find a way to let go of their sexual energy or begin to crave relationships with people outside of their immediate circle. If there is ongoing marital discontent, one or both partners may start to exhibit signs of depression.

Accusing and Combating: People who are starved of sex may become resentful, aggressive, or spiteful. They may argue about the lack of sex with their spouse. One partner may experience intense guilt or think they're acting improperly if the other doesn't show any sexual interest.

Adultery: It's possible that you or your partner is so dissatisfied with your marriage that you seek out sexual fulfillment from people outside of it. In these situations, one may experience jealousy, mistrust, or divorce. If certain behaviors are not consensual, bad feelings could arise even in an open relationship.

HOW TO REVIVE A SEXLESS MARRIAGE

You may be able to bring your marriage closer together and resume having enjoyable, frequent sex. You might be able to revive the passion and excitement in your romantic life by using the advice below.

Discover Why Your Marriage Is Sexually Vapid: It might be necessary to identify your partner's sexual issues before addressing them. The problems may not be obvious or they may have nothing to do with sex or sexual activity. Even in a happy marriage, emotional distress, sexual health problems, or recurrent arguments, for instance, can make it difficult to establish a physical connection. You might be stopping sex because of stress in other aspects of your life, such as work or raising children. This could also be having an effect on your relationship. In cases where the reason for the lack of intimacy is not evident or bringing up the topic seems too much to handle, a couple's counselor can facilitate communication and uncover any hidden issues between the couple. See a doctor for assistance with sexual dysfunction if your health problems are interfering with your physical intimacy in a low- or no-sex marriage.

Focus on Communication: In relationships, effective communication can involve more than just words. It might also be essential to use nonverbal clues, and each partner might need to develop the ability to communicate while keeping their spouse's emotions and mental health in mind. There are lots of resources available for couples who have trouble communicating effectively. To better understand how each of you expresses and receives love and affection, you and your partner might find it helpful to take the love languages quiz. Another option would be to use a workbook on constructive relationship techniques.

Adopt a Kind/caring Approach: It's unlikely that accusing and blaming your partner will boost their sex drive or make them feel more interested in having sex. Your sex life and relationship may be healthier and happier if you and your partner are able to respectfully and kindly communicate your needs and desires. Think about discussing the relationship as a whole. Try saying, "I think this would be fun for us," as opposed to, "I want to try this." You can gain a deeper understanding of your partner's viewpoint by being receptive and attentive to their conversation. Inform them if there is anything they would like to try that you find uncomfortable. One essential component of a happy relationship is consent.

Handle Inherent Conflicts: Sexual conflicts may be an obvious symptom of a deeper, more persistent issue in your relationship, even though they may also be the cause of some marital problems. It might be essential to address any underlying problems in order to rebuild a healthy sexual relationship. Addressing these suppressed feelings may help you if you or your spouse holds any grudges or resentment against one another. Recognizing, affirming, and resolving low self-esteem issues together can help to improve your relationship if you or your spouse experiences them.

Look into Other Options for Intimacy: Consider exploring non-sexual forms of intimacy if one partner finds sex bothersome or if there is a lack of sexual intimacy. For instance, you could write each other love letters, hold hands more frequently, or share a kiss before work. According to a medically reviewed study, couples' level of relationship satisfaction was influenced by their perception of intimacy and enjoyment during kissing.

Seek Alternative Channels for Your Passion and Energy: You may find happiness and solace in other forms of expression if you are in a sexless marriage or relationship, or if one partner wants sex but the other doesn't. Taking up a new sport or hobby can improve wellbeing and help release stored up energy. It may be easier to bring up the subject of intimacy with your partner when you're more at ease. You might also experience relief from masturbating and self-stimulation. When one or both partners have sex with someone other than their spouse, it's common for couples with different libido levels to choose an open relationship.

Engage in Sexual Activity without Contact: It can be beneficial for couples to enjoy each other in different ways if they believe that their lack of sexual activity has rendered their marriage sexless. If you typically only try penetration, for instance, you may try oral sex, playing with toys, or acting out a fantasy. To test how long they can go without having sex, some couples may try making out or kissing for extended lengths of time. Others could read up on new positions or play a game like sex dice. Sometimes, one or both partners' dissatisfaction with your current sex patterns can be the cause of a lack of intimacy and a low desire to have sex in the future. You and your partner may feel more fulfilled and eager for sexual intimacy if you can discover new techniques for achieving arousal and orgasm.

CAN MARRIAGE SURVIVE WITHOUT SEXUAL INTIMACY?

Yes, sexual intimacy is acceptable in a marriage. But only in the event that neither party is interested in having sex is this feasible. There's a chance the marriage won't last if a couple doesn't seek assistance from a sex therapist or counselor if one partner has low sex drive or if one partner is asexual. This is particularly true if the foundation of the relationship was shared sexual experiences rather than an emotional bond or friendship.

It is entirely up to the two individuals involved in the relationship to decide whether to stay and try to make their love life work in spite of the sexual dysfunction. You might think about joining a support group for men in sexless marriages if you want your marriage to succeed even after an unsuccessful attempt at intimacy.

CHAPTER THREE

ROUTINE OF COUPLES WHO HAVE GREAT SEX

They Restrict Pornography: For certain couples, erotica in books or photographs can intensify the mood in the bedroom. However, a heavy addiction to pornography can make it difficult for some men to achieve an erection and have an orgasm with their partner. Additionally, porn creates false expectations about what real sex is like. That may undermine their partner's self-worth and cause relationship problems.

Their Definition of Sex Is Broad: Sexually satisfied couples typically realize that having sex isn't the only thing that matters. Additionally, research indicates that they typically have at least one intimate encounter per week. Maintaining a routine isn't a recipe for happiness right away. However, developing a close physical relationship with your partner can often indicate that things are well between you.

They Are Not Fixated on Orgasms: sexual climaxing is not the aim of every sexual experience. It can put a lot of strain on certain partners. Building closeness with your partner just requires sensual touches or any other kind of connection that suits both of you.

They have faith in one another: According to studies, couples who lie about what they enjoy and don't enjoy doing in the bedroom are more likely to experience discontent. Thus, let each other know if you're having problems achieving an orgasm or if your libido is lacking. Inform your partner if anything makes you uncomfortable or if you feel self-conscious about your appearance.

They Create Time: Your body takes longer to react to sexual stimulation as you get older. An erection can be more difficult to achieve and maintain in older men due to lower testosterone levels. Women may experience dry vagina and delayed arousal as a result of a decrease in estrogen during menopause. Make an effort to allot enough time for each other to enjoy sex.

They Exchanged Words: Fulfilling sex can be greatly aided by knowing where your partner's sexual "starting point" is. Some people, mostly men, can get into a mood without any prompting. Some require a cue to become aroused, particularly women. You can both be happier if you accept those differences.

They Make Contact: Making physical contact with someone is a great way to foster trust and connection. Sensate focus is a technique used by sex therapists. This exercise investigates your feelings toward various types of touch. Additionally, it lessens the pressure to achieve a sexual "goal" like penetration or an orgasm. Sensual touch exercises can bring couples closer together and enhance the enjoyment of intimacy.

They Acquire Knowledge: Sexual bliss can be equaled with knowledge. Your sex life can reach new heights when you get to know each other's physical erotic zones, what turns you on, and how much stimulation you need.

They Seek Counseling: Through touch exercises, education on arousal and desire, and improved communication skills, sessions with a certified sex therapist can help with intimacy issues. Talk therapy might help your relationship as a whole if your problems are the result of other problems.

They Look for Accomplishment: Perfectionism comes from practice: Your body's response pathway that facilitates easier arousal is strengthened and built up when you engage in activities that elevate your feel-good endorphin levels, such as physical activity, laughing, creating art, or having sex.

They Provide for Their Partners: Studies reveal that happy couples are in the sack when they prioritize their partner's satisfaction and enjoy each other's company. You may find yourself acting out your partner's sexual fantasies or engaging in sexual activity more frequently than you usually would.

They Create Time: Your body takes longer to react to sexual stimulation as you get older. An erection can be more difficult to achieve and maintain in older men due to lower testosterone levels. Women may experience dry vagina and delayed arousal as a result of a decrease in estrogen during menopause. Make an effort to allot enough time for each other to enjoy sex.

They Make Use of Tools: Some may perceive using lubricant to relieve dryness or using a pillow to prop themselves up during sex as an acknowledgement that they require assistance in order to arouse their partners. However, the reverse is also true. Your experience will be better if you pay closer attention to both your partner's and your own comfort.

They Put It to Use: It might sound like a deal breaker. However, University of Toronto researchers discovered that happier intimate relationships are shared by couples who think that having a great sex life is a result of hard work and effort rather than finding a soul mate.

They Continue to Be Flexible: Sex is not normal. Everyone has different preferences, varying levels of desire, and varying degrees of importance. Age, physical health, and the stresses of daily life can all have an impact on your libido and priorities over time. A more fulfilling sex life is often the result of a couple remaining open-minded and flexible about their sex needs and feeling better about themselves.

WHAT IT MEANS TO MEET A WOMAN'S NEEDS IN BED

When you go into a woman's bedroom, how can you make her feel satisfied each time? How can we improve her sex experience? How can one please a woman? The knowledge of what it truly means to satisfy a woman provides the answers to all of these queries. To put it simply, satisfying a woman entails being aware of her needs and desires during your most private interactions with her, attempting to meet them, and doing so in a courteous manner with her permission.

Not being egotistical in bed is another requirement for satisfying a lady. Recall that being an excellent partner in bed is more about your ability to read your partner's needs and navigate her body than it is about your size or endurance. It shouldn't be too difficult to figure out how to make sex better for her if you return her efforts to make the experiences enjoyable for you and don't just concentrate on your fulfillment.

Knowing how to emotionally satisfy a woman is another crucial factor that many men miss when concentrating on sexually satisfying a woman. Recall that men and women approach and perceive sexual intimacy in different ways. Women view sex as a more emotional experience than men do, who view it as a more visually driven process. Your sexual connection is likely to be better the more emotionally connected she feels to you. Nevertheless, evidence suggests that there is no universally accepted definition of female orgasms and sexual pleasure. One woman's solution might not work for another. But if you and your partner communicate honestly and openly, it's nothing you can't get the hang of.

Just ask your girl if you want to know how to make her feel good in bed. And then be willing to modify your sex strategy to meet her needs. You could, for example, ask her for advice on how to have better sex and approach it precisely the way she prefers. That should increase her pleasure quotient, which would raise your both of your arousal levels and improve your sex experience.

FOUR MAIN EFFECTS OF SEX ON THE BODY

Four separate phases of sexual arousal were discovered by sex researchers William Masters and Virginia Johnson in the 1960s, each with its own physiological implications. Following their research, these four categories are now widely used to explain sexual response:

EXCITATION OR DESIRE: The tissue in the clitoris, vulva, pelvis, vagina, and penis fills with blood during the desire phase. This makes the nerves in these body parts more sensitive. Additionally, transudate, a fluid produced by this blood flow, lubricates the vagina. The body's muscles start to contract. Because of the increased blood flow, some people breathe more quickly or experience skin flushing.

PLATEAU: An individual's level of arousal keeps rising during the plateau stage. Increased sensitivity is felt in the clitoris, penis, and vagina. During this time, changes in sensitivity and arousal may occur in a person. Interest and arousal may fluctuate in intensity and decrease.

CLIMAX/ORGASM: An orgasm may occur when the right stimuli and mental conditions are met. The quickest and most efficient route to an orgasm for the majority of females is clitoral stimulation. It's the only way to an orgasm for some people. Males may require extended stimulation of the penis' head or shaft. A male orgasm typically results in ejaculation, though this is not a must for an orgasm to occur. Some females also ejaculate during an orgasm; however, scientists are still debating what exactly is in this fluid.

During an orgasm, males and females alike experience severe contractions of their muscles. These contractions occur in the rectum, penis, and pelvis in men, and in the vagina, uterus, and rectum in women. Certain individuals report having contractions all over their body.

RESOLUTION: The body gradually returns to its pre-arousal state as the muscles relax following an orgasm. Males and females go through this process differently. Many females experience an orgasm immediately after ejaculating, while most males do not. Most males and many females go through a refractory phase during the resolution stage. The individual won't react to any form of sexual stimulation during this period.

CHAPTER FOUR

SEXUAL COMPATIBILITY

Great sexual compatibility is when two people are on the same page regarding their physical desires, kinks, and other physical characteristics and are having a healthy sexual life and sparkly chemistry. Is there more to sexual compatibility than just that, or does it stop there? Is it enough to meet your sexual match and call it a day, or do you keep trying? Louisa, who dated Drake for four years, claims, "We were incredibly physically compatible, but he needed to move cities and put his career first, so he wanted to take a year off from the relationship."

When we first met a year later, we were drawn to each other magnetically. This is a sign of sexual compatibility that only occurs when you have strong chemistry with someone. We became aware of our sexual compatibility during our year apart. We weren't committed to one another, but we also didn't feel like going to bed with anyone else. It goes without saying that the reunion was incredible. We are a sexual match made in heaven!

Love, emotional, and intellectual closeness are prioritized in long-term relationships, but sexual compatibility is also a crucial factor that is frequently disregarded. Is it better to marry for compatibility or love? We would say "both" in response to this frequently asked question because developing a solid and healthy relationship requires both.

WHAT IS SEXUAL COMPATIBILITY?

Strictly defining sexual compatibility is difficult because different people have different standards and preferences. However, in general, having great sex does not equate to being sexually compatible. When your preferences in bed align, your moods coincide, and your sexual drives are similar, you are considered sexually compatible. When both partners are willing at the same time and don't start fore playing and then say they'd rather go to bed because they're too tired, you know you have a compatible sexual relationship. Naturally, being moody or exhausted once in a while doesn't necessarily indicate that you two aren't compatible sexually, but if your chemistry is strong, your vibes will generally converge.

WAYS TO DETERMINE IF YOU ARE SEXUALLY COMPATIBLE

YOU HAVE SIMILAR VIEWS ON SEXUALITY: It does feel like this when you and your partner have a sexual relationship. Whether you enjoy traditional, kinky, or even just plain old-fashioned public sex (just make sure it's somewhere clean!), you have a sexual compatibility. You can agree on the frequency and duration of sex, the type of relationship you want (open or monogamous), the type of environment you like, and the things that make you feel attracted to each other.

YOU ANTICIPATE THINGS SIMILARLY: Having similar expectations regarding sexuality is essential for sexual compatibility. You've discussed your boundaries and know what to anticipate when your partner asks for sex, but you're also excited if they surprise you. You follow the current and have fun while doing so. During an orgasm, you don't care about your performance or the face you make. (We promise—no one has a particularly attractive orgasmic face. aside from their spouse). All you want is to enjoy yourself and give and receive pleasure in your own special ways.

YOU PRIORITIZE FULFILLMENT: Assume that although your partner detests PDA, you two don't really disagree on anything when you're in the bedroom. So, are you compatible sexually? You are, indeed. There will inevitably be some topics on which you cannot agree. You are physically compatible as long as you are giving in bed and are committed to making each other happy, even though he may prefer doggie fashion and she may prefer cowgirl.

YOU EXPRESS YOUR NEEDS: Sexually compatible couples maintain open lines of communication throughout their partnership. In your 20s, you may find something appealing, but by your 40s, it may have completely changed. However, you are sexually compatible when you both accept how your bodies and desires change together, which occurs when your preferences change together. It's vital to have sex conversations. That could be something you do after the act, or even while you are performing it. Your partner would adore hearing, "I just loved that new thing you did today."

YOU SHARE SIMILAR INTERESTS: You are sexually compatible if you both enjoy having sex on the kitchen table as well as the bed, if it doesn't matter if the lights are on or off, and if you occasionally enjoy getting dirty in the backseat of your car. When you enjoy cuddles and agree that kissing is healthy, or when you prefer to spoon and have private conversations over fully engaging in sexual activity and you feel completely fulfilled by the intimacy, then you are also sexually compatible.

HOW NOTABLE IS SEXUAL COMPATIBILITY IN UNIONS?

The cornerstones of a healthy relationship are sexual compatibility, communication, respect, love, and understanding. A couple may believe they are sexually compatible in the beginning of a relationship because they have certain chemistry. However, after getting married, they might eventually come to the realization that their libidos are mismatched and that, although one of them values sexual intimacy above all else, the other believes that a basic level of intimacy in a relationship is sufficient.

How does it feel to have a sexually compatible relationship with your partner? It takes time for a couple to figure out whether they are sexually compatible, though sometimes this can be accomplished with minor compromises and discussions. In general, one indication of sexual compatibility is feeling at ease with your partner on a sexual level. When you are with your partner and feeling comfortable in your sexual position, you stop worrying about the stretch marks on your thighs and the paunch you are gaining. You feel completely accepted by your partner and at ease in both your body and mind.

"Sex is far more important when a couple is young, maybe in their 20s, than it is when they are in their 40s," says sexologist Dr. Rajan Bhonsle, MD, Hon Professor, HOD, Department of Sexual Medicine, KEM Hospital and GS Medical College, Mumbai. They are content to engage in other activities at that point since they have other priorities in life, such as their kids, investments, and travel. Both partners find that their sexual lives have a more comfortable rhythm and are content with it. In terms of sexual compatibility, both partners must feel the same way. According to the sexologist, some couples who are in their 60s or 70s still have wonderful sex, and the only things that make this possible are matching libidos, mutual understanding, and a certain level of comfort.

According to Dr. Bhonsle, a couple's sexual compatibility is determined by two factors: their level of desire and their physical ability to give and receive pleasure from one another. According to Dr. Bhonsle, "a couple may have comparable physical desires, but the man in the relationship may find it difficult to maintain an erection for an extended period of time, so the desire is not complemented with fulfillment."

What can you do to improve your sexual compatibility with your partner? According to Dr. Bhonsle, who holds diplomas from the American Board of Sexology and the American College of Sexologists, "People take the help of a sexologist to achieve that compatibility because they understand how important it is to have a sexually compatible partner." In a loving and understanding relationship, mismatched libidos—such as when a wife wants to have sex once a week while her husband wants it every day—can be worked out and sexual dysfunction treated.

Additionally, according to Dr. Bhonsle, there are happily ever after sexless marriages. There's nothing wrong with a couple having their fair share of satisfying sex in their youth and moving on to other pursuits in their 40s if they no longer want to have sex. However, the sentiment must again be reciprocated. Another sign of sexual compatibility is when neither of you is interested in having sex at the same moment. It is not possible for one partner to be uninterested while the other is; in that scenario, the marriage could serve as a fertile ground for an extramarital affair.

HOW TO KNOW YOU ARE SEXUALLY COMPATIBLE

Actually, this is a million-dollar question. Some individuals confuse compatibility with immediate sexual chemistry. However, once the novelty wears off, something that was enjoyable for two or three sessions may not remain so. When two people are prepared to make concessions and engage in compromises, as well as when they are open to discussing what works and what doesn't, they are considered sexually compatible. "It could happen that you find little common ground with a person during a conversation but when you are between the sheets you see that you match instantly," says dating coach Cora Boyd, who is based in Seattle. In a relationship, the indicators of sexual compatibility will be present. It only requires that you recognize those cues and trust your gut.

YOU SAVOR THE MOMENT AND NEVER KEEP TRACK OF THE MINUTES OR HOURS: It's highly unlikely that you will be able to respond when asked how long you've had sex. You have never measured your sessions; therefore, what was important to you was their quality. When your levels of desire are similar and you can spend all day in bed on a Sunday, but still manage a quickie in the morning on a workday, you are sexually compatible. You simply enjoy being physically intimate with your partner, and it doesn't really matter how long you've engaged in this behavior.

YOU'RE STOMACH TREMBLES WHEN YOU LOOK YOUR PARTNER IN THE EYE: Sure, romance novels are known for this tendency, but even fiction has some basis in reality. You and your partner are experiencing sexual tension outside of the bedroom if your stomach flutters whenever you look at each other. There's benefit to this. Is it normal to get butterflies in your stomach when you see your significant other during a party?

Do you still feel this way after spending a few years with your partner? It indicates that throughout the years, you have managed to maintain the spark in your relationship. For you, what does compatibility feel like? It evokes the same kind of closeness as when you cook together, hike together, or find yourself in between the sheets with your significant other.

YOU EAGERLY ANTICIPATE MAKING LOVE:

Do you also have sexual thoughts about your partner when you think of them? Do you find yourself mentally repeating what you did this morning in bed? Would you like it to occur once more? This indicates that you have strong sexual chemistry as well as sexual compatibility, both of which will contribute to a long-term satisfying relationship. You don't consider a movie star or the hot guy next door to be the best; instead, you tend to fantasize about your partner. That is, for the most part. You are completely content with your partner in bed because you believe they are the only person you need to satisfy your sexual fantasies.

Be aware that it is unrealistic to expect perfect sexual chemistry or compatibility. There may be days and nights when one partner's sex game is a little off, even if you two are completely in sync sexually. However, your expectations of the tenderness and messiness of the sex are reasonable. You look forward to it.

YOU HAVE CONCERN FOR YOUR PARTNER'S ENJOYMENT: When you're both thirsty, Boyd advises you to make sure your date gets a glass of water for themselves or for the two of you. This reveals a lot about their character. They probably wouldn't give a damn about your enjoyment in the bedroom if they were egotistical. Generous individuals in bed are those who are considerate of their partner's pleasure in and out of the bedroom. Compared to someone who is solely interested in their own pleasure, it is easier to be sexually compatible with someone like this.

YOU'RE OPEN TO MAKING CHANGES: The state of sexual compatibility is not always automatic. You must put effort into it. For example, one partner may enjoy being kinky while the other may find the idea repulsive. To get the most out of their relationship, two people in that situation might be open to trying new things and making some adjustments. In bed, two people will inevitably disagree on everything. Recognizing that and talking about it are crucial.

YOU ACKNOWLEDGE THAT BAD DAYS WILL OCCUR: It makes sense for you and your partner to realize that no two days will be the same. It's possible that you've had a very busy day with the kids and that he's under stress at work. So, is a hug and some kisses enough for you? Sexually compatible couples are very understanding of one another's circumstances and refrain from pressuring a partner into having sex when they are not ready. Some days he might not have the best erection, or she might not have the best lubrication. Sexually compatible partners acknowledge this, frequently joke about it, and avoid letting their tension escalate over their differences.

YOUR CONSTANT GOAL IS TO INCREASE THE PLEASURE OF THE SEXUAL EXPERIENCE: You strive to increase the pleasure of having sex. When you have some free time, you should watch some YouTube videos that let you try out different foreplay positions. To improve your sex lives, you both frequently read articles online or consult books like Kama sutra. You want to improve your sexual life and take it seriously. To experience the romance on screen that you can bring into your bedroom, you and your partner may occasionally watch porn or films like The Notebook, Blue Lagoon, or 50 Shades of Grey together.

YOU CONSIDER THE METHOD RATHER THAN THE CONCLUSION: If your sexual chemistry is compatible, you will find that experiencing physical intimacy is enjoyable in and of itself; the climax is never the main attraction. On some days, you could just relax on the couch and watch Netflix, and on other days, you could plan to have sex in the shower. Enjoying the atmosphere of doing it in the shower or on the couch, you can't help but laugh when you trip over the shower head or fall off the couch. Making love is something you enjoy doing completely.

YOU ENJOY EXAMINING EACH OTHER'S BODIES: Your partner, and you yourself, will know things about your body that you are unaware of when you are sexually compatible. You both really enjoy examining each other's bodies and locating the erogenous zones and pleasure spots. Furthermore, you feel satisfied if your discoveries bring them joy. Getting to know one another's bodies' takes time. For asexually compatible couples, it's a joyful journey of exploration. This indicates that you are compatible sexually if you are doing it frequently.

THERE IS STILL A SEXUAL ATTRACTION OUTSIDE OF THE BEDROOM: Even when you are out on a dinner date with someone, you will know if you are not having a sexual connection with them. When you look at each other, the sparks will not fly. However, if you are attracted to someone sexually, you may get shivers from your partner's intense gaze while candlelight dances across their face.

Beyond the bedroom, sexual compatibility is important. You can sense the sexual attraction when you simply hold hands while he drives or when she puts her hand around your waist while you are taking a selfie. In certain situations, you can get excited just by being near your significant other in a closed area like a smoking room or elevator. On your way to work, you might smell their perfume and spend the entire day planning what you would do to them once you got home.

WHAT TO DO WHEN THERE IS NO SEXUAL COMPATIBILITY

Most of the time, sex is explored after a couple falls in love. They may consider the love, understanding, and emotional closeness in the relationship when they discover they are not sexually compatible, believing that sexual attraction is merely one aspect of it. It wouldn't be catastrophic if you didn't have it. However, Dr. Bhonsle asserts that in the long run, sexual incompatibility may become a problem. He cautions, "Sexual incompatibility is sometimes the reason marriages fail." The other positive elements of a relationship may be destroyed by sexual incompatibility, which can cause resentment, frustration, and bitterness.

The good news is that by working on it, one can develop sexual compatibility. To find out how to get better at having sex, you could visit a sexologist together with your partner and have a direct conversation. You could look inward and see that if you both could work things out and come to a better understanding, rather than viewing your sexual incompatibility as a lost cause and seeking sexual fulfillment outside of the marriage.

Sexually incompatible couples occasionally choose to swing together, pursue open relationships, or lead polyamorous lifestyles. Regardless of the decision they ultimately make, they should remember that sexual compatibility is a crucial component of a healthy relationship and should not be disregarded. You can also ascertain compatibility with the aid of premarital counseling. However, in most cases, sexual compatibility can be worked around, a middle ground can be found, and long-term sex can be enjoyed when there is trust, care, and clarity in a relationship.

CHAPTER FIVE

WOMEN'S HOTTEST EROGENOUS ZONES

Sensual foreplay does more than you might think for increased sexual pleasure. Furthermore, exploring a woman's body in addition to the obvious turn-on spots may add more spiciness and pleasure. There are many erogenous zones on women, which can be stimulated to instantly arouse them sexually. Setting the mood for amazing sex can be as simple as feeling her erogenous zones and exploring her body.

The body of a woman is an amazing place. "Women cannot be turned on like faucets, where everything flows out with just a single turn." It demands more work. Women cheered when Twinkle Khanna said this at coffee with Karan. It is true that way. The need for pleasure in women is somewhat minimized because of the overwhelming male perspective on erotica and sex. Though little is known about what makes women tick, they are objectified in movies, fashion shows, and advertisements. If it's discussed, it happens in private and amid a lot of laughter. The surprisingly most erogenous zones for women are being revealed, along with some hidden information about them.

HER HAIR: In every sexual play, the hair is a boost. Samson's strength is entirely derived from the hair on his head, as Deliah was aware. The way you touch a woman's hair, however, says a lot about you. Because you are intimate with them, women prefer that their hair be noticed, even though it is completely hidden when they are out in public or dressed up. You can gain brownie points if you kiss her and run your fingers through her hair at the same moment. You can let her know what you like by giving her a little tug while she's lying down on you. However, if you hold onto her hair and gently tug it as she approaches the climax, she will always be appreciative.

HER LIPS: Everyone is aware of this one. Generally speaking, we aim for it first. A well-placed kiss can make or break a relationship for many women. Thus, don't rush things. Delay the inevitable; take your time. Gently touch the corner of her mouth and plant a gentle kiss on her lower lip. Await her greatest moment of desire, and then give her a deep, moist kiss.

HER EARLOBES: You can use earlobes for more than just earrings. Own and assert them as a sensual location on your woman's body. It's meant to be occasionally nibbled and even bitten. Giving pleasure yields receiving pleasure. Identify her tender points in and around her ears. Use your tongue to follow the path until the entire earlobe is in your mouth.

HER NIPPLES: For some, a black band covering the nipples is sufficient to pique their interest. Nipples are the place where women are supposed to bite. They don't really care for a soft suck or a light lick. However, avoid nipples at that time of the month. During your menstrual period, you don't want to aggravate your already sensitive and painful nipples.

HER NECK: The area that women find erogenous is also a vampire's preferred bite site. Approach from the back, gently press your teeth to the spot, and feel the shiver go down her spine. Wrap one arm around her waist, the other around her shoulder, and proceed with the attack. Make her want it by tease and tempting her, and then gently bite her to feel her melt in your arms. It's also the ideal location for a love bite.

HER NAVEL: It's very enjoyable to play with the navel; some people feel tingly, while others feel aroused. Lick it, smell it, and listen for her reaction. Giving someone a kiss on the navel can never go wrong. Have you ever attempted to lick your navel? At least not in a proper way, those who have not sampled wine from a woman's navel have not made love yet.

HER CERVICAL REGION (SPINE): Remember the spine if you want to witness her arch in a pleasurable way. Women's spines are extremely sensitive. They adore being kissed or stroked down the spine. If you caress it while kissing her, it truly sends a chill down her spine. Alternatively, you could go in the opposite direction, climbing her from the back and kissing her all the way up her spine before biting into her neck like a vampire. To maximize her pleasure, while you are inside her, run your nails smoothly up and down her spine.

HER CLIT OR CLITORIS: When it comes to a woman's sexual pleasure, the clitoris is the star. Apologies, that isn't penetration. One cannot overlook the peculiar structure located directly above the vagina: the clitoris. After you locate it, don't let go of it. She can become delirious with pleasure with a tongue tip or a firm thumb press on the clitoris. Remember this as well: rub lightly and listen to her whimper and moan in blissful ecstasy.

HER KNEES: Knees pose a challenge. Others may feel it better in their right knee, while still others may feel it more in their left: As you spoon her, find out which one it is. You can determine which way to go by using a gentle fingertip touch. As you kiss them, maintain eye contact and hold both of their knees in front of you. With every kiss and lick, watch how her expression changes. She will recline her head and savor your touch as you observe.

PROVEN WAYS TO SATISFIED HER IN BED

Teamwork is the key to good sex. Recognizing this fact at all times is the first step in learning how to make a woman feel good in bed. Although it may be true that sex is a basic human need, approaching the experience from the standpoint of making love to a woman can make it much more joyful and healthful. Without realizing that foreplay is essential to giving a woman a satisfying sexual experience, men frequently rush the act. Your woman isn't necessarily ready for the act just because you guys are fired up. You will be well on your way if you adopt a laid-back demeanor and give her wishes some thought.

Take your time getting to know her body, experimenting with various foreplay positions and novel experiences that make her feel good if you want a fulfilling and healthy sexual relationship. Until she's ready, put the piercing sex on the back burner. Additionally, when you do manage to get her to orgasm during sex, try not to push yourself too hard. Or believe that, as a result, you lack the sexual skills necessary to win a woman over.

She frequently experiences an orgasm during foreplay, and she might or might not have another during sexual activity. Actually, studies show that men experience penile-vaginal penetration orgasms more frequently than women. Furthermore, only 31–40% of women can experience an orgasm during a sexual encounter by themselves. That was one myth dispelled! In the end, you just need to concentrate on making it enjoyable for both of you in order to satisfy your woman every time you have sex. You don't need to stay longer or work harder. With these suggestions on how to impress a woman, we're going to show you exactly how to achieve that:

TO WIN YOUR WOMAN OVER, LOOK PRESENTABLE AND SMELL GOOD: Setting the stage for successful sex requires good hygiene. Take a shower, brush your teeth, and put on a light perfume before going to bed. Ensure that all facial and body hair has been cut or removed. Observe your underwear carefully. Regardless of how long or new the relationship is, maintaining poor personal hygiene can turn someone off right away. Don't get comfortable with this. Any progress you may have made in picking up new tricks and tips to entice her can be undone by making such mistakes in bed. Long-term partners and spouses frequently grow so accustomed to one another that they cease making an attempt to woo and impress one another. What makes so many men wonder, "How do I figure out how to sexually satisfy my wife/girlfriend?" is this complacency in a relationship.

START OFF WITH A KISS: To start with a kiss and let things develop from there is one of the most crucial foreplay strategies. Don't limit yourself to giving her French kisses or just lips-to-lips kisses. The majority of women enjoy receiving kisses on their necks, breasts, and other erogenous areas like their toes, inner thighs, and shoulders. Every woman has different erogenous zones, so you'll need to explore her body to find out what energizes your partner the most. Kissing a girl all over her body can give you sexual pleasure. Make sure this foreplay tip is at the top of your list if you're looking for ways to improve sex. Yes, giving a woman the perfect kiss at the perfect moment and intensity can be the best way to satisfy her in bed.

EXTENDED FOREPLAY WILL BE EXTREMELY BENEFICIAL WHEN YOU PLEASURE YOUR WOMAN: Good foreplay is your best ally if you're wondering how to get your wife excited in bed or how to arouse your girlfriend/partner sexually. The secret to pleasing a woman is to build her up gradually. Women have amazing bodies as a blessing. There is plenty of room for investigation. In F.R.I.E.N.D.S., Monica gives Chandler a seven-point formula that he can use to solve the puzzle of how to satisfy Kathy, his former girlfriend. That's precisely the goal you ought to pursue as well. To really get her fired up, take your time, mix things up, and do the 1 to 7 dance rather than making it quick and hurried.

To arouse her, you must, in essence, become an expert at foreplay. This is going to work like magic, but take your time before you penetrate her. Consider incorporating some roleplaying into the mix to kick things up a notch while you're at it. You could get yourselves some exciting and fun costumes that will heighten the tension and make your act last longer, or you could order her some sexy lingerie.

IN BED, ACT LIKE A GENTLEMAN: You may wonder how to make her feel good in bed. We only have one word to say to you: consent. Regardless of the phase of your relationship, you should always prioritize getting informed and enthusiastic consent. Recognize the distinction between abuse and passion. Avoid going too far and hurting her feelings. Making love to a woman should never turn violent; instead, it should be a hot, passionate, and enjoyable experience for both of you. Establishing sound sexual boundaries and getting her permission are the best ways to guarantee her comfort. Press pause right away if your partner appears uncomfortable at any point. No implies no.

Rather than assuming that you know your way around her body and are giving her the time of her life, the easiest way to make sex better for her is to ask her what she likes or if she is enjoying what you're doing, read her body language cues, and follow her lead. For your partner to fully let her guard down and enjoy the experience, she must feel secure with you.

SPICE UP YOUR SEX LIFE WITH SOME DIRTY TALK: Understanding how to arouse a woman's mind as well as her body is essential to successfully engaging in sexual pleasure. Try your hand at some dirty talking to see if you can satisfy her in bed. But also in this situation, exercise caution and respect for sexual boundaries and consent. Try not to overdo it so much that she feels dehumanized and unappreciated. Conversely, discuss with her your likes and dislikes, your attraction to her when you see her nude, what you would like to do to her, and other topics.

Even worse, you can make your regular sex entirely new by making her happy with some dirty dancing. Sexual relations take on a new and refreshing appeal when this happens. Becoming happy in bed is the goal. A woman can be greatly gratified by feeling wanted and desired, and being wanted sexually is a very flattering experience for her.

SOFTLY WHISPER SWEET NOTHINGS DEEP INTO HER EARS: Recall our earlier discussion on how it's critical to be able to emotionally satisfy a woman in order to establish a sexual connection? Whispering tender words that reassure her that you love and care for her is one way to ensure that her emotional needs are satisfied during your most private moments. Make a seductive comment while you nibble her ear. Hit her with a few sensual lines as soon as you've kissed her. Turn her on by bringing up her sexual fantasies. Continue to look her in the eye while you're at it. This will make her extremely lustful. Finding the perfect pressure point to pique a woman's interest is just one aspect of the art of seduction. The true art of seduction often originates from the mind and doesn't always happen in the bedroom. Perhaps it's time to start thinking outside the box if your goal is to impress her with your moves.

TO PLEASE YOUR WOMAN, GET DOWN ON HER: Try surprising her with oral sex after you've spent a fair amount of time on foreplay. For her, this is far more fun than even intimate sex. The best way to please a woman is to orally stimulate her during sex, and there are many tips for doing so. Take a cue from the movie

Fifty Shades of Grey and give her a good licking, biting, playing, grabbing, and all of that! Unexpectedly giving a BJ can make her reach previously unheard-of levels of pleasure. That's just how impulsive BJs really turn the heat on for you. It's important to take your time and not rush things, to reiterate. You won't ever have to worry about how to make your girl feel satisfied in bed if you do it correctly.

LICKING AND TAUNTING YOUR WOMAN WILL MAKE HER HAPPY: One of the simplest ways to satisfy a woman in bed is to play with her body and run your hands over it. Touch her gently and give her a few tickles. Give her a breast massage or give her some downtime. Remember to tease her effectively with your tongue. Your woman will react wonderfully to these moves and a little bit of licking will work wonders. Watch her sigh with pleasure as you gently bite the creases in her skin. Reaching these climax points for women will immediately turn up the heat and result in incredible sex. In addition, there are a number of entertaining goods and toys that can enhance the enjoyment of using your tongue to explore her body. To make every pore in her body come alive with excitement, you can, for example, sprinkle flavored kissing dust all over her body and lick it off.

TRY A QUICKIE: You probably already know that there isn't a single right way to woo a woman. You need to be open to experimenting with various approaches and methods of sex in order to be able to genuinely ignite the sexual connection. Never running at full speed is not the goal. When trying to give a girl a sexual pleasure, the element of surprise is fantastic. It can be really satisfying to catch her off guard (and in unexpected places), and it can also result in an incredibly sultry session afterwards.

It's possible that she's working on a task when you give her a passionate kiss. She would be gasping and pleading for more as things quickly get out of control. Feeling wanted and witnessing their partner lust for them and never be able to get enough of them are two essentials for women to have happy and healthy sexual lives. A quickie that says, "I've got to have you here and now," perfectly captures all of this. Naturally, you want to convey your passion and desire, but you also want to be careful not to violate her consent in the process.

INQUIRE ABOUT HER PREFERENCES: Do you want to learn how to make your partner, wife, or girlfriend feel lustful? Just put an inquiry out to her. Allow her to share with you what brings her intensity and desire rather than forcing your will on her. Give precedence to her wants and needs over your own. Consider the things and methods she finds pleasing. In a relationship, being generous with your sex is crucial. Along with providing basic answers to your queries about how to completely satisfy a woman in bed, this will assist your woman in letting go of her inhibitions. Allowing a woman to take charge could be one of the keys to her satisfaction. Inform her that you will simply follow her lead and that she is in control. Ask her to use words and/or deeds to communicate to you where she wants you to be or what she wants you to do. She will reveal her favorite things to you when she assumes a dominant role in sex, and it will also assist her in letting go of her inhibitions and embracing her sexual urges.

TRY MAKING LOVE IN VARIOUS LOCATIONS: Get out of the bedroom and explore the kitchen, study, and even the bathroom, among other areas of the house. To feel that rush of adrenaline, you could even try having sex outside. The change of scenery and pace will be welcome; a little sex adventure keeps things feisty in the relationship. If your interactions with her are getting predictable and boring and you're not sure how to make it better, you might want to think about having a quick vacation. Finding a lovely hotel or resort in the area, making a reservation, and spending the weekend away from it all with just a change of clothes, underwear, and sex toys will allow your sexual life to blossom into a passionate experience.

TO MAKE THINGS INTERESTING, USE SEX TOYS: Even though you may think you're the best at making love, we recommend using sex toys to stay at the top of the game. A vibrator is a great way to get your woman really excited. It will only make women feel more pleasurable in bed. Do sex toys improve relationships? We believe that they are! In addition to traditional sex toys such as vibrators and dildos, you can enhance the pleasure by using leather whips, foam foreplay mats that interlock, and nipple rings and clamps. These can increase arousal in ways you never would have thought possible when applied to the pressure points for female orgasm. These strategies and tactics for foreplay have the power to really elevate your sexual connection.

ACTIVATE YOUR FANTASIES TO MAKE YOUR WOMAN HAPPY: Find out what her greatest dreams are, and then make an effort to realize them. When you two realize those wild dreams come true, things might get more sensual. This is a fantastic method to combat relationship boredom. Naturally, you should only consent to things that you are totally comfortable with; otherwise, it might cause more harm than good. Getting her to orgasm each and every time you have a sexual encounter—ideally several times—is the ultimate tip and bonus. Do not forget that greater is better. Just penetrating sex is rarely enough to cause women to orgasm, as we have already discussed. Either make her get to the big-O before or after the sex to ensure she doesn't miss out on her fair share of the fun. Make the necessary decisions, but don't abandon her.

CHAPTER SIX

COUPLE'S BEST SEX POSITIONS WITH DIAGRAM

Should you possess prior experience in a committed relationship, you are aware that it is usual to experience a loss of the initial chemistry you shared during the courtship stage. Even though there are many benefits to a partnership, such as the fact that you are likely familiar with your partner's physical attributes, maintaining the romantic chemistry, particularly in the bedroom, may require some additional effort after a certain amount of time has passed.

With enough repetition, even a tried-and-true sex routine between you and your partner can become stale. Fortunately, you can bring back the romance in your relationship by experimenting with various sex positions that allow for lots of extra kissing, touching, whispering, and making eye contact. It's crucial to be upfront and honest about your sexual needs before attempting a novel coital arrangement. There's a myth that 'The One' can read minds. Setting the mood deliberately can also have a significant impact. Romance can be greatly enhanced by even small actions like blocking out time on your calendar, lighting candles, dressing in your best clothes, and taking a soothing bath before sex.

You'll be able to stay in the bedroom longer and enjoy yourself more with these sex positions. Sex with a partner can be especially stressful if you are among the one-in-three men between the ages of 18 and 59 who experience premature ejaculation.

- Will you experience an orgasm too soon?

- Is she going to be let down?

It has the feel of a crapshoot, only with you as the only shooter. Thankfully, there are exercises like the squeeze technique, Kegels, or stop and start methods, as well as desensitizing sprays like Promescent that can help, especially in the long run. But what many men fail to understand is that the way you have sex can affect how quickly you orgasm just as much. In order to help you stay in bed longer, let's look at the top sex positions with diagram.

SPOONING POSITION

How to Carry It Out: With your front pressed against her back in the spooning cuddle position, both partners lie on their sides. She is the little spoon, and you are the big spoon. Your partner needs to slightly spread her legs apart. Using your hand, locate her vagina and enter her from behind.

How Beneficial It Is:

- You won't be able to make the long, wild thrusts that push most men past the point of no return in this sex position because your strokes will be very short.

- It's a great stroke for her because the short strokes target her G-spot.

- Consider using your fingers to stimulate her clitoris while concentrating on grinding your hips against her butt.

- It's easier to feel good about your own orgasm whenever it occurs if you can make her experience one.

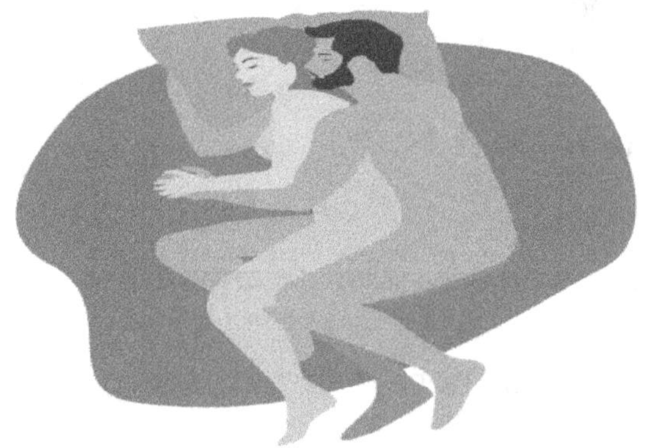

COWGIRL POSITION

The Method: Lie on your back, Lean forward and let your partner mount you, then straddle your hips and insert your penis. Then, she can mount your penis like a bullfighter on a cowgirl.

How Beneficial It Is:

- Giving up some control can really help you in this particular sex position.

- Your ability to thrust quickly and forcefully, if the spirit moves you, is taken away from you because your partner has nearly total control over the penetration.

- Make sure your partner understands that you should focus on her pleasure and limit your own.

- Most likely, this will entail clitoral stimulation and deep grinding, which is the ideal way to break your penis.

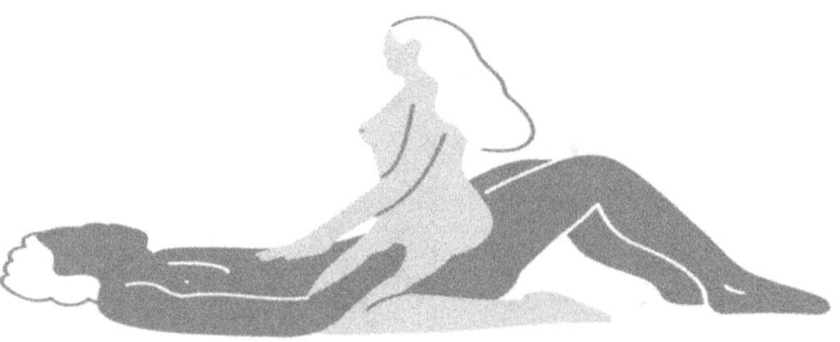

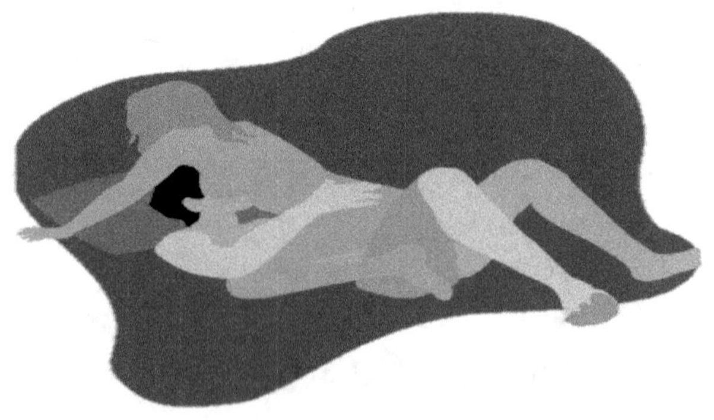

INVERTED COWGIRL POSITION

How to do it: While the receiving partner straddles their hips and faces away from their partner below, the penetrating partner should lie on their back. The person at the top can lean forward to make eye contact and intensify the intimacy. Furthermore, showing your partner your butt is a very private moment.

"For one thing, many women (in particular) might feel body image concerns about their butt," Queen says. "To show it off can be an act that takes some nerve and can feel somewhat vulnerable, and that can open up feelings of intimacy if we're received by the other person in a way that supports the risk we took."

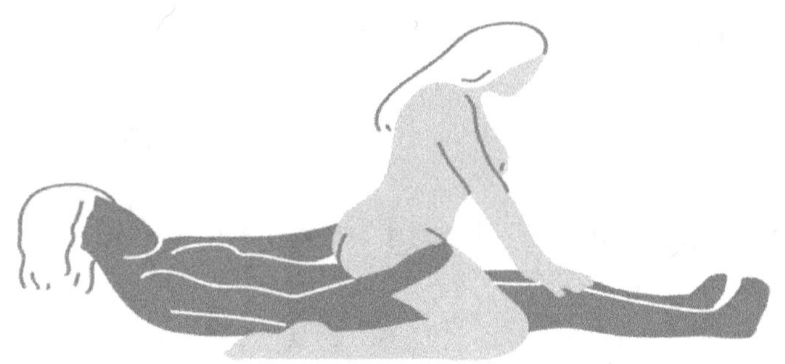

THE LEADING WOMAN POSITION

How to Carry It Out: The woman climbs on top of you, just like a cowgirl, but she lies chest to chest, like a missionary in reverse.

How Beneficial It Is:

- This posture limits his ability to thrust while enabling the woman to completely encircle the penis.

- Without forcing you to lose control, she can relish the intense sensation of fullness and grind her clit against your shaft.

- Since she is in charge, make sure to let her know when you need a break and are getting too close.

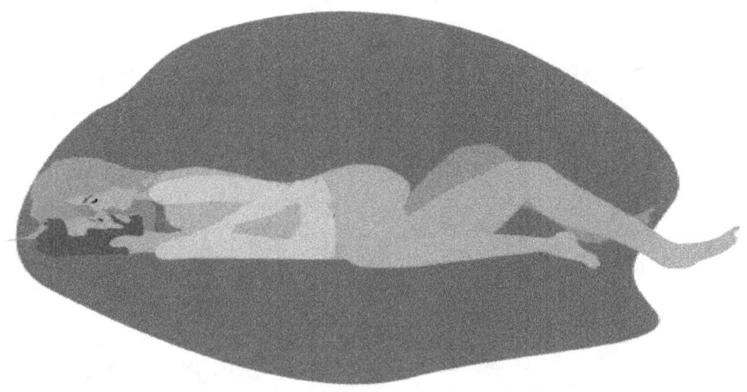

THE YUM YAB POSITION

How to Carry It Out: The woman faces him and straddles his hips so that he can enter her from the front while the man sits on the floor or bed.

How Beneficial It Is:

- One of the advantages of this position is that it is difficult to hold.

- The man is unable to hold himself and his partner in place while thrusting arbitrarily.

- It's an extremely private position that's perfect for winning your partner over and learning from her responses.

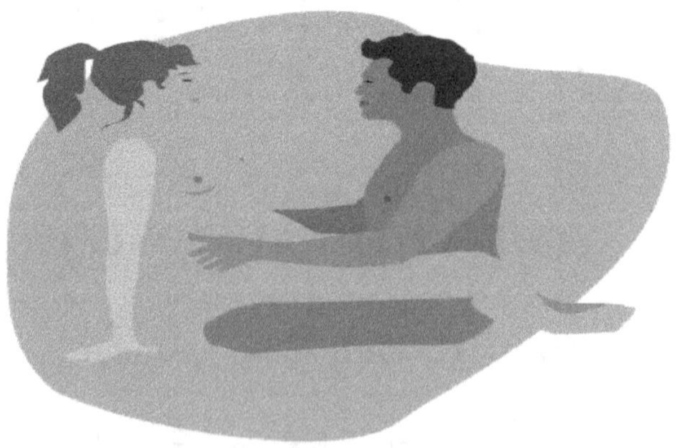

THE SALUTE IN STANDING POSITION

How to Carry It Out: Locate a nice, cozy pillow that she would be comfortable lying on. Ensure that the pillow is positioned close to her lower back. He must stand facing her and toward the bed or table in order to engage in sexual activity.

How Beneficial It Is:

- He can thrust quickly or slowly in this position, which allows for deep penetration and intimacy as well as a great opportunity to take a break if necessary.

- She will benefit greatly from this position because the pillow will lift her pelvis slightly, enabling deeper penetration and better targeting of her G-spot.

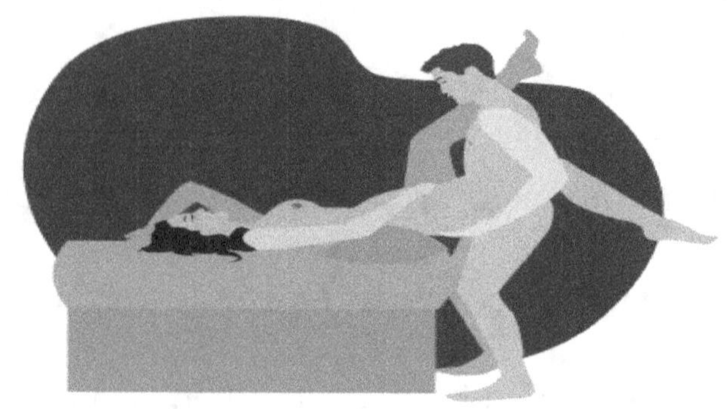

BALLET DANCER POSITION

How to do it: For this one, the penetrating partner raises one of the receiver's legs instead of completely supporting their partner. The receiver is more stable in this manner. If you want to make things sultry or impromptu, Hall continues, you can do this against a wall, on a counter, or on a table. You can't go wrong because you're essentially copying your favorite romance book.

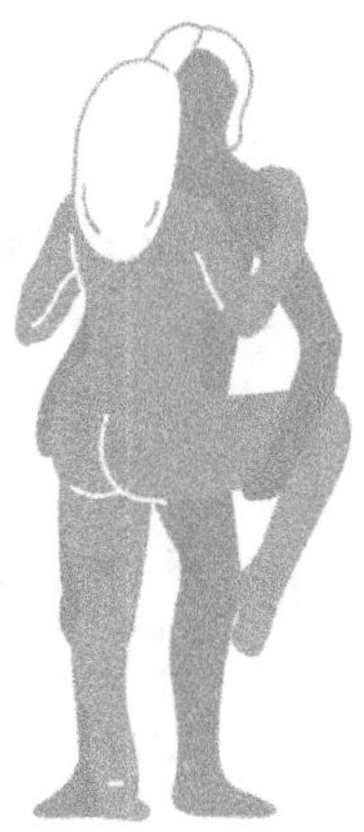

IN PARALLEL/SIDE BY SIDE POSITION

How to Carry It Out: Spooning is comparable to this, but partners face one another. Your partner lifts the free leg and wraps it around your hip while you are face-to-face on your sides, allowing your hips to access her vagina.

How beneficial it is:

- The depth to which each partner thrusts is controlled by them both, making the sex position both active and passive for both parties.

- The man gives up some control, which limits how much he can thrust and lets him concentrate on sensations.

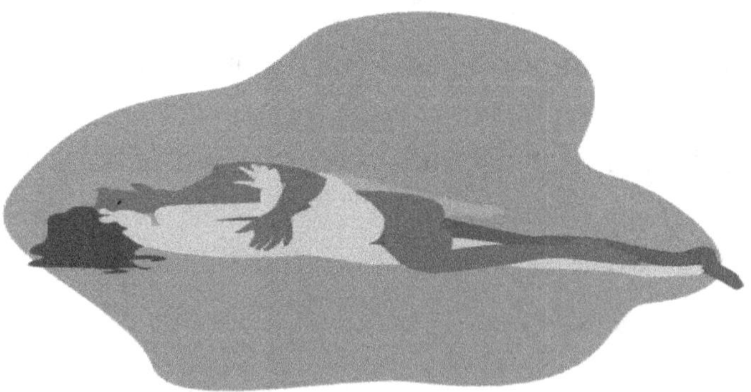

MISSIONARY GRINDING POSITION

How to Carry It Out: Because you are the one doing all the thrusting and have access to deep penetration, the missionary position is one of the easiest to lose control of. By forcing you to press your penis deep and remain there while grinding your hips against hers, the grinding missionary completely reverse the dynamic of the situation.

How Beneficial It Is:

- It's simpler to prevent your penis from becoming overstimulated when there aren't the lengthy, powerful thrusts.

- Your partner will enjoy the front-action grinding in the interim. It rubs her clit while filling her vagina fully.

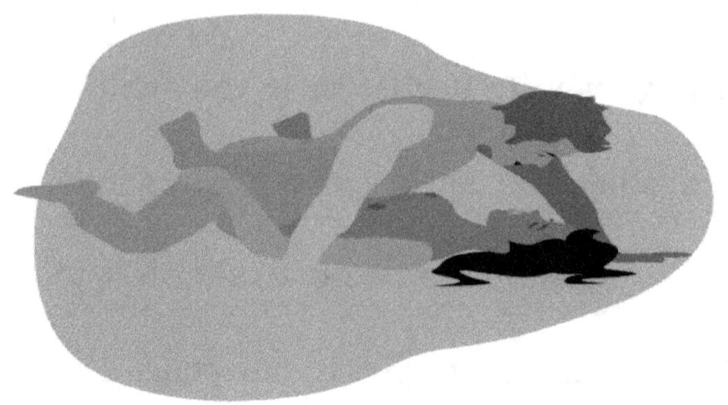

MISSIONARY POSITION

How to do it: The penetrating partner should place themselves between the legs of the receiving partner, who should lie on their back. One of the simplest sexual positions is missionary, and it's a classic for good reason. It's one of the most intimate positions there is, with lots of close contact and eye contact. "It's easy to make missionary more intimate because you're face to face,

Eye contact, kisses, and seductive words of gratitude, she continues, can all heighten the romance of the situation.

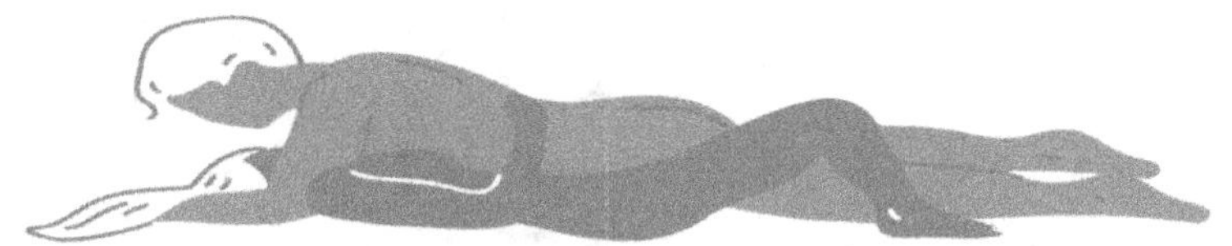

DOGGY STYLE POSITION

How to do it: The penetrating partner enters the receiving partner from behind while holding their hips. The receiving partner then goes to all fours. There are still ways to make it more intimate even though you won't be there in person for this one. A kiss on the jaw or neck can be given by the penetrating partner leaning in. Another option is for them to remain nearby and whisper in their partner's ear.

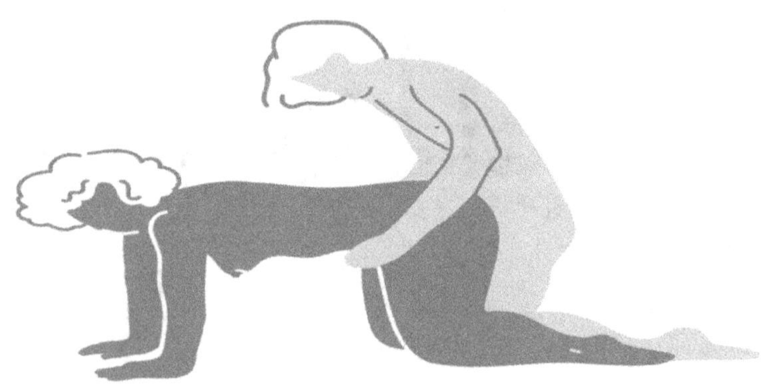

GET ON YOUR KNEES POSITION

How to Carry It Out: With her legs spread wide, your partner lies on her back in the missionary position. You enter her missionary style from a perpendicular position, kneeling upright.

How Beneficial It Is:

- Without the leverage of your free hips, you are unable to thrust as forcefully or deeply from this position.

- Additionally, you have control over the situation and can lower the intensity if necessary.

- Additionally, the strain needed to keep yourself kneeling can take your mind off your pleasure to the point where an orgasm is postponed.

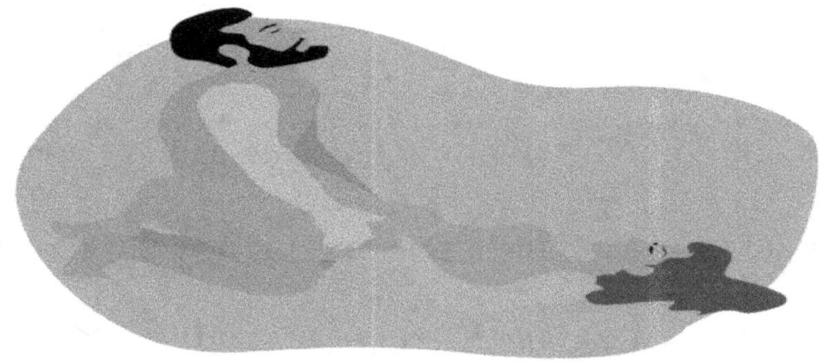

POSITION OF THE SEASHELL

Method: This is for you if you have a great deal I mean, a great deal of flexibility. The recipient partner reclines, crossing their ankles behind their head and lifting both legs as high as possible. The penetrating partner continues from there as they would in a missionary.

Due to the high degree of flexibility required for this role, the penetrating partner can really bring the romance factor by seeing to it that their partner is comfortable. For instance, they can check that the pillows are perfectly positioned or that they feel supported. "This is a face-to-face position that allows for kissing and eye contact, and it makes it easy for the partner on the bottom to touch both themselves and their partner.

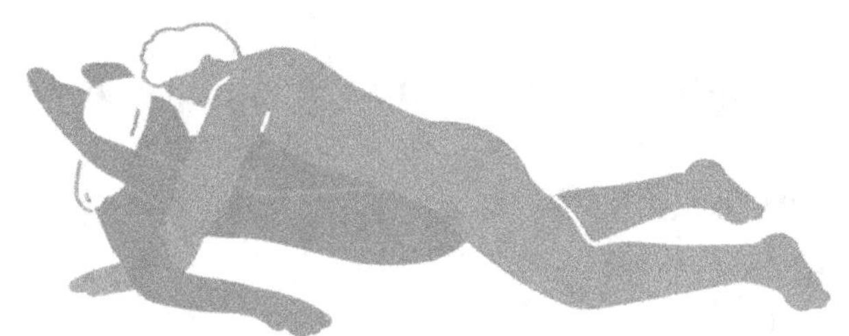

OCCUPY THE THRONE POSITION

How-To Method: Her back should be to you while she stands, and she should lower herself onto your lap and insert your penis in the process. You should sit on a chair and supervise her.

Why It's Beneficial:

- The woman is in charge and will often grind against your hips, relishing the slow, deep penetration without thrusts that are too quick or aggressive.

- Though she does enough squats at the gym, she may bounce a little.

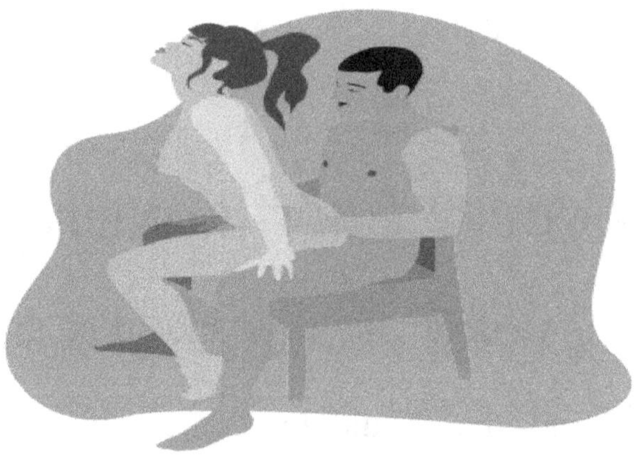

DEEP MUTUAL MASTURBATION POSITION

Technique: Select a cozy location opposite or adjacent to one another, and then alternately engage in individual or group masturbation. "I always like to say that sex does not always have to include penetration," Hall asserts. "One of the most intimate acts that you can do together is mutual masturbation."

By telling your partner the truth about what pleasure means to you, you are communicating with them during mutual masturbation. Both ways, it gives your partner very specific instructions on how to make you happy.

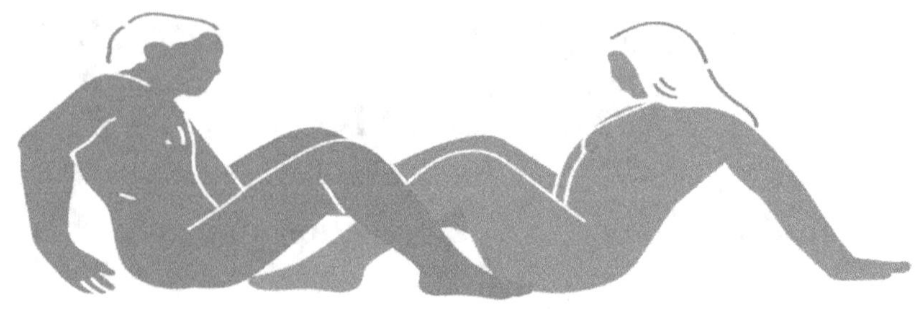

HOW SEXUAL POSITIONS MAKE YOU LAST LONGER

Many men are simple beings. All they are familiar with are two or three sexual positions. Premature ejaculating men are unaware that certain sexual positions can actually prolong their climax for a variety of reasons.

- *To keep you from getting overstimulated, they don't permit thrusts that are as deep or prolonged.*

- *They don't rely on any penetration or thrusting, which slows down the rate at which you get aroused.*

- *You focus more on keeping the position than on the sensations in your penis because they are hard to execute.*

- *They provide you the power to decide how much stimulation you get and prevent you from going over the edge.*

- *They put her pleasure first, which usually entails less forceful thrusting than you might imagine.*

He becomes considerably less monotonous in bed and is not constrained to the same two positions by discovering the ideal positions for him to stay in longer. Women value the chance to experience novel feelings. It can be exciting to never know what to expect from you in bed.

IMPORTANCE OF CHANGING POSITIONS DURING SEX

Women adore the total porn star move of switching positions during sex because it gives your sex positions some variety and fresh sensations. Changing positions implies something completely different for men who ejaculate prematurely: a chance for a break if they sense the big finish drawing near.

You can experiment with twelve new sex positions from this article to see if you can extend your time in the bedroom. It could be very alluring to go crazy and switch positions every 30 seconds in an attempt to postpone your orgasm and impress your partner with how amazing you are.

Variety is something that women adore, but they also enjoy the opportunity to settle into a position and experience whatever feelings it brings. Too many position changes could make her feel like a prop in your own intimate sexual decathlon. Change things up, of course, but exercise self-control. During a sexual session, four or five positions are sufficient.

WAYS TO SWITCH POSITIONS WITHOUT BREAKING THE GROOVE

You probably picture sex as sensual and elegant in your fantasies. However, in practice, the physicality of sex can often leave one feeling a little clumsy and even confused. Fortunately, part of the fun is figuring out how to move during sex so as not to ruin the mood. Your sexual encounters can take on a new dimension when you use slow, sensual, and rhythmic motions.

First and foremost, it's critical to keep in mind that there is no right or wrong way to move during sex. It's not fun to try and ignore your own feelings in order to live up to some ideal of sexiness. Give it some time to explore, figure out what your body responds to, and then keep doing it. You must follow your own instincts and decide what kind of movements' suit you best, whether they are soft or a little rough.

Having said that, there are a few tips that can improve your sex and pleasure levels. **One thing to bear in mind is rhythm.** This is already second nature to some people. But if you're not a trained musician or dancer, it might take some getting used to maintaining the rhythm. However, there's a simple fix. Your Tango says that when you're having sex, put on some music and let the bass move your body. This will assist you in moving rhythmically, steadily, and smoothly. (There are many sex playlists available that you can play when the time is appropriate if you need assistance.)

There may occasionally be a pause in action when moving between positions. According to the Women's

Health website, if you want to maintain the rhythm, try utilizing sex moves that naturally flow into one another. For example, a simple leg sweep can turn cowgirl into reverse cowgirl, and a simple backward lean can turn seated into missionary. You can try different combo moves with your partner until you find one that works for you.

One more piece of advice: **move slowly.** For example, as stated on the Cosmopolitan website, when you're on top, try moving your body in extremely slow motion forwards, backwards, and sideways. (I don't mind if this advice sounds like it came from an R&B song.) You can discover what feels good without getting tired by using soft, flowing motions. Feel free to move even faster or slower after you're in the correct frame of mind.

Finally, move in a way that, whatever that means to you, **makes you feel sensual.** Perhaps you have the hips of a belly dancer. Perhaps you roll your body. Perhaps you simply run your hand down your partner's back. The whole experience can only be improved with an occasional extra touch. Go outside now and experience a newfound appreciation for your body.

WOMEN'S DESIRES FROM MEN

FACTORS THAT COULD ALTER THE INTIMACY SCENARIO: Understanding what women want from men is one problem that has always existed in romantic relationships. Men often don't realize what their partners expect from them, which causes a lot of relationship problems. Especially considering that there are a lot of things that every woman wants her man to do without her having to ask. These silent, unfulfilled expectations gradually accumulate into a heavy weight that has the power to destroy your relationship, especially when men have no idea what they are. Communication can only go so far on this front because most women find it difficult to express these hidden desires in a relationship. Getting to know a woman's inner workings and what she needs from a man is your best chance. Every woman is different, of course, but generally speaking, what she looks for in a man falls into one of the ten categories listed above.

Action between the sheets is not what we mean specifically when we talk about intimacy. Intimacy can take many different forms, even though it is a crucial component of any relationship and the intimacy between couples. Every partner should strive to develop each one in order for the relationship to be well-rounded. We are here to support you if the classic what women want from men is impeding your progress in this area. Women first and foremost desire a closer, more meaningful relationship with their partners at least the great majority of women. Reaching that doesn't require big gestures, expensive presents, or showy celebrations. Enhancing your intimacy can be as simple as learning the most enjoyable things to do with women. Similarly, you two can become closer than you can ever imagine if you try to establish a connection with her outside of sex.

Getting the fundamentals of a romantic relationship right is the key to understanding what women want from men. The following qualities are desirable in a man, so start with them and work your way up based on your partner's expectations and the particulars of your relationship:

MAKE AN INVESTMENT IN PILLOW TALK: Although having sex is wonderful, have you ever tried just talking while lying next to your partner and holding their hand? You'll see how well it works to develop emotional intimacy between you two if you try disguising sex for a late-night conversational session. These pillow chats can reveal new facets of each other's personalities, from childhood tales to reminiscing about the early years of your romance, sharing your feelings and informing your partner about your goals, fears, and hopes. Give it a shot, even if you believe you know everything about each other from your lengthy relationship. You would be pleasantly surprised to discover how much more you can discover and get to know about your companion.

BREAKFAST IN BED FOR HER: Do you want to increase your intimacy even further? You can accomplish that goal in a big way by doing something as easy as occasionally bringing her breakfast in bed. Surely, one of the things that every woman wants her man to do on his own initiative is this. This show of affection and concern shouldn't be reserved for holidays, birthdays, or anniversaries. It's the ideal moment to get in the kitchen and make her something healthy and delectable on any lazy morning when you both have some free time.

Pancakes, sautéed veggies, grilled sausages, and cheese don't have to be served in an elaborate fashion. It works just as well to have something as basic as eggs and toast with juice or coffee.

DEVELOP IT: Beyond a fast buck, women desire more. We understand and amazingly sex is good. However, it's not the best idea to go through the entire process quickly as though you have a deadline to "finish." More, much more, is what women desire than a fleeting bang. Make love to her whole body, not just the part that pique your interest, is one of the sexiest things you can do to a woman. "Foreplay is probably the best bit," remarks Ramona, a mid-30s woman who has been involved in sexual activity for more than ten years. The most crucial aspect of foreplay, according to her, is a lengthy kissing session, which is closely followed by a lot of touching and leisurely undressing. She describes it as "like a chorus," meaning that you can't help but return to it. She is also very specific about the fact that she wants her partner to "judge the pace of...touching" and "know when to offer the tongue."

GET HER CLITORIS WELL PLEASURED: The best sex occurs when a man can locate and satisfy his clitoris. Every woman can't get enough of this one thing in bed. It's what they all want. It's regrettable, then, that most men have a tendency to ignore what will surely drive their women insane. According to Angelina, "sex is best for any woman when the man knows how to find and pleasure the clitoris." Many women assert that when it comes to orgasms, good tongue-on-clitoris action has frequently produced more consistent results than penetrative sex. Angelina continued by saying that she finds it extremely sexy when her partner approaches her slowly from behind, his arms loosely wrapped around her waist and his fingers caressing her clitoris. That is not to say, however, that a woman needs this specific quality in a man. You can investigate, test, and determine what suits you and your partner the best. But if you want to deepen your relationship with the woman in your life, pay attention to the seductive C.

SPEAK ALL DIRTY OF HER: You're in for a pleasant surprise if you believed that talking dirty and verbalizing your craziest sexual fantasies is something that only men wanted to do. Women also desire this from men. Even the best foreplay can't always make a woman feel more attracted to you than a little dirty talk. No, the dull conversation you hear in pornographic videos is not what we're discussing. What these women considered sexy was not a "You like that, huh?" It's especially sexy, says Azel, an erotica reader and writer on occasion, to have her man kiss her and whisper in her ear all the things he wants to do and the sequence he wants to do them in while his hands "go places."

DON'T FAIL TO HIT HER G SPOT: Your partner may not be as interested in getting intimate as you are if you feel that things are not progressing as quickly as you would like. This could be because you enjoy your sex more than she does. It could be due to our inability to locate and activate the elusive G-spot. Rosette, a successful young lady who is in touch with her sexuality, isn't afraid to tell us that her boyfriend has a penis that is on the average side. She does, however, adore the fact that her partner can make good use of it and accept his size. She is very vocal about the significance of "hitting the G-spot" and talks about how his slightly arching penis is ideal for her in missionary and cowgirl roles. The G-spot, which is a few inches inside the vagina and on the front wall, is said to be a very stimulating area.

One of the top ten qualities that every woman looks for in a man is undoubtedly his ability to find her sweet spot. Try searching for a little bit of texture on the otherwise smooth front wall of the vagina if you're a man and are having trouble finding it.

HUG AND CONVERSE: Attention is what every woman looks for in a man. Therefore, avoid, at all costs, the urge to turn around and head back to bed after a productive session. For a woman, it can be very disappointing and off-putting, and it could give the impression that you're reclusive and distant. Your post-coitus habits may be the reason behind accusations that you're only interested in sex if you've ever experienced them. One easy habit can make all the difference in the world: after the act is over, simply talk to her for a while while holding her in your arms.

Even if you're exhausted from your sleep or anxious about waking up early the following day to ace that crucial work presentation. And never forget that it's strictly forbidden to look at your phone right after an orgasm. These seemingly innocuous behaviors not only ruin the romance and prevent you from becoming intimate with your partner, but they may even contribute to her turning against you.

INVESTIGATE HER SEXUAL/EROGENOUS ZONES: Different places can make a woman squirm with pleasure and turn her on. Working a woman's erogenous zones until she begs you to stop but still wants more is one of the most enjoyable things you can do to her. Women may differ in these areas, but everyone undoubtedly has more than a few. A woman can be turned on and made to squirm with pleasure by various places and spots, such as the earlobes, navel, tops, and thighs. It's your responsibility to identify your woman's weak points and take advantage of them for mutual gain. We guarantee that you won't turn back.

BE ARDENT: Feeling wanted and coveted is what women most want from men. What could be more fitting than indulging in passionate lovemaking to elicit that feeling in her? No matter how long you've been dating, avoid falling into the routine of dragging your partner around for sex. At that point, any chance of developing intimacy in your relationship is lost, and the spark actually goes out of the relationship.

Try new things, venture, and discover as much as you can in the bedroom. Don't, however, end there. Sex is not always a necessary correlate of passion. It works wonders to keep the romance going and your bond strong to grab her and give her a passionate midday kiss. Your partner will feel closer to you than ever if you make frequent expressions of your longing for her a part of your life.

The desires of women for men are not all that complicated or dissimilar from those of men for women. The one thing that sets women apart from men is their desire for a deep emotional bond in a partnership. You should contribute equally to creating and maintaining that relationship as a partner, both inside and outside the bedroom.

CHAPTER SEVEN

OUTDOOR SEX FOR COUPLES

All it takes to have outdoor sex is the two words that define it. You try something new and daring by having sex outside or in a public place rather than on your regular bed. When it comes to sex, going public can help you break out of your routine and add a wild, sensual, and seductive appeal to the same sex. And once you realize how much fun outdoor sex can be, you might start looking for outdoor sex spots frequently! Throughout your life, you have probably encountered a number of sex experts who have provided you with a wealth of sensual advice, ranging from tricks to make your partner scream with pleasure to playful yet seductive bedroom antics. And as long as you are inside the guarded walls, all of those suggestions would be effective.

However, how would you feel if someone told you that having sex outside would really make it even more enjoyable? Yes, that sounds amazing. It's also true in reality. Even the most boring couples can have their desires sparked by a seductive outdoor makeout. Until you give it a try, wait. Here are some reasons to remove the game from your bedroom.

JUSTIFICATIONS FOR HAVING OUTDOOR SEX

✓ ***Become sexually confident:*** Sometimes, you and your partner sense something is lacking in your sex, but you are unable to identify it. You have attempted both conventional and unconventional sexual positions, but without success. Perhaps having sex outside is all you need.

✓ ***Wonderful sexual experience:*** Now, not only the physical location, but also your partner has left a lasting impression on you, all of the romantic spots you visited during your honeymoon or travels have a particular place in your memory. Your memories of sex are no different. Why not experiment with outdoor sex in various settings to add more unforgettable experiences?

✓ It can be exciting and stimulating to have sex outside of the bedroom because you are trying to avoid being caught while also feeling hot and bothered. Sex is elevated to a whole new level by the pleasure and danger of being discovered, and you get to experience some incredibly creative ways of making love. What else could make you feel lustful if that doesn't? We give you five reasons to try having sex outside, and we know you'd want to do it even more after reading them. A popular sexual fantasy is to have sex in a pool or beneath the stars. After all, who wouldn't want to? It's simple: having sex outside should be on your bucket list since it's a popular sexual fantasy.

✓ ***To take a chance and try something daring:*** The thrill of having sex while running the risk of being caught in the act intensifies the pleasure. Outdoor sex is your ideal game if you've always been one for excitement and thrills.

✓ ***To break up the monotony of bedroom sex:*** Do you not think that the backdrop, curtains, and sex location are always the same? What would it feel like to have sex in a different setting? Something that is exhilaratingly adventurous in addition to being exquisitely set. Consider it.

CONSIDERATIONS FOR OUTDOOR SEX EXPERIENCE

No matter how experienced you are at outdoor sex or whether you are a novice couple looking to try it out, keep these pointers in the back of your mind at all times.

Choose wisely where to have your outdoor sexual encounters: You don't want to be prodded by a police stick, bothered by obscene passersby, or worse, have your intimate moments captured on camera by pornographers. Additionally, check if the weather is conducive to having sex—snowboarding might be too intense.

Always try a different location to ensure that people are not growing suspicious of you and to maintain the excitement. Each time you test it, move it to a new location.

Always arrive ready: To avoid awkward situations, carefully consider where you want to have outdoor sex and come prepared. Take the example of always bringing a padded mat for sex in areas with potentially uneven flooring. Keep first aid supplies, condoms, and lubricants in your sex-aid kits.

When dressing for sex, choose items that are simple to put on and take off. Avoid wearing intricate clothing that could be difficult to take off and ruin the entire experience.

Refrain from breaching the law: It is considered offensive and illegal to expose one's privates or engage in lewd behavior in public. Choose a secure location or use tact to ensure that your outdoor sex is covered.

TOP LOCATIONS FOR OUTDOOR SEX

It can be an exciting move if you have chosen to take your game outside of the boundaries. However, there are good and bad places to have sex outside. If you choose the wrong place, you could end up with serious consequences, bug bites, or being nude in public. Thus, you should consider your options carefully before having sex outside. You can essentially choose any location beneath the sky. But you have to try these public places for sex. And keep in mind that it will be an experience of a lifetime.

THE ROOFTOP: Have you ever tried it? It seems like something out of a romantic film because of the wide open area, the breeze, and the stargazing that comes afterwards. Go up to the roof, but only do so when the weather permits.

INSIDE A CAVE: Find a cave on a hilltop or beside a stream, and like our ancestors, get close to one another. It's an exciting place to have sex outside.

THE ELEVATOR: I believe that the elevator is more in love with you than it is with you. This location is inherently captivating. How about the risk? Absolute value

A DESERTED BEACH, you and your companion perched atop each other, and the gentle sound of the waves crashing ashore. Could it get any more exciting and wild?

UNDERWATER: Possibly in the swimming pool? While having sex underwater can be very exciting, we should exercise caution because the condom could come off. Also, you might require lubricants.

ALL-ADULT MUSIC FESTIVAL: Try outdoor sex at this place if you're searching for a little bit of glitz and glamour. Campsites are available at most music festivals so you can pitch your tent and get started.

THE LONELY NOOK OF THE LIBRARY: Nearly all couples are drawn, for some reason, to having sex in a library that is off limits. Couples are actually drawn to this location more because of the morality surrounding sex.

SAUNA: The saunas in most public clubhouses and community pools are seldom used. It is possible to have sultry, hot sex.

THE BACKYARD: According to sex therapist Kat Van Kirk, it's probably a good idea to try outdoor sex somewhere nearby if you're new to the idea. Go for it! Locate a place in your backyard that is private and that your neighbors cannot see into.

TAKE A BACKSEAT AND STOP MUTTERING IN THE MOVIE THEATER: For couples worldwide, it is typically a preferred location. Yes, the entire notion of having high-up seats in corners

OPEN FIELD: You should absolutely stop and play for a while if you happen to come across a sizable area of open field when traveling. In the fog, having sex outside is insane.

THE AUTOMOBILE/CAR: If you've watched any porn or movies, you're aware that one of the most exciting spots for outdoor sex is the back of a car. Particularly when it begins to rain. Yes, all of those dreamy, romantic movie scenes are playing right now!

A BOAT: A sailing boat has the power to energize any couple; however, be mindful of the weather conditions. It adds to the excitement if the sex becomes a little shaky. But avoid getting seasick.

THE AIRPLANE: The real source of exhilaration and high altitude, Maybe the bathroom.

THE ART MUSEUM: For sophisticated people who want a retro feel for their outdoor encounters. Find a corner with little foot traffic and start burning some steam.

IN A TENT: If you're camping and staying the night in a tent, go ahead and enjoy some filthy games, just don't go overboard and knock the tent down.

High school students do act in ***OPPOSITION TO THE TREE,*** but the appeal is still the same. As he works on you, wrap your legs around his body and work those thighs hard.

THE WOODS: Do you and your companion enjoy going camping? Then you ought to definitely try having sex in the wild in the woods. But be careful not to get bitten by insects or bugs, and perform the task while standing.

CHAPTER EIGHT

FOODS THAT IMPROVE YOUR PERFORMANCE AND YOUR SEXUAL LIFE

WATERMELON: Citruline is an amino acid that is abundant in this juicy fruit. It is converted by your body into another amino acid that helps relax your blood vessels, arginine. In the same way that Viagra treats erectile dysfunction that can stimulate blood flow to your sexual organs.

SPROUTS/SPINACH: This isn't typically considered a seductive vegetable. However, it can increase your sex desire in a number of ways. Magnesium, which is abundant in this leafy green, can raise testosterone levels.

It also contains iron, which, especially in women, can support arousal, desire, orgasm, and sexual satisfaction.

THE OYSTER: These days, oysters aren't just a fancy food item found at a few select restaurants; they're also increasingly common at seafood restaurants and other regular eateries, where they're served as a condiment with other main courses. Zinc is abundant in oysters and contributes to overall vigor. An additional benefit is that it increases testosterone production. Thus, it contributes to increasing your libido and sex drive.

AVOCADOS: Avocados are highest when eaten raw because they are high in antioxidants. These go well with salads, but you can also eat them on their own however you like. The greatest thing about avocados is that they are an excellent source of potassium, oleic acid, and vitamin B1. These benefits include strengthening your testicles and increasing your energy, which in turn improves your performance in bed.

WALNUTS: All that these nuts are edible seeds that come from pine trees. They are typically added as a side dish or as a topping for dishes that include chicken, meat, or fish and serve as a complimentary dish to the main course. They can be added to salads as an ingredient as well. Pine nuts have numerous health benefits, including a significant reduction in erectile dysfunction in men and an increase in sexual desire in women, both of which lead to fantastic sex between the partners.

CHOCOLATE: Aphrodisiac qualities are well-known for chocolate, and dark chocolate is particularly well-known for its ability to increase libido. It increases serotonin and phenylethylamine production, which is beneficial for people who have low libido. It also boosts your libido. Chocolate can improve your libido and sexual arousal.

EGGS SOFT-BOILED WITH THE YOLK STILL INSIDE: Saturated fats and cholesterol are the two main substances that are known to increase the production of sex hormones like testosterone and decrease the production of cortisol, the main stress hormone. You can regularly eat eggs as they are a good source of HDL cholesterol. These are good cholesterol that are very healthy for your body and increase your desire for sex.

POMEGRANATES: After being cracked open, the pomegranate's hard shell contains seeds that are packed with nutrients that improve blood flow and stimulate the body's arteries and veins. They also include substances called polyphenols and vitamin C. All things considered, they support heart health and help prevent high blood pressure. They boost blood flow to the heart, brain, and other essential organs and provide you with energy! As such, those who regularly consume pomegranates exhibit improved responses to sexual stimulation and foreplay in bed.

ENTIRE GRAINS: These consist of specific types of cereal for breakfast in the morning and oatmeal. You read that correctly! Eating whole grains and oatmeal on a daily or regular basis helps to increase the amount of testosterone produced in your bloodstream, which improves your sex life tremendously. Thus, stop rolling your eyes when you see your cereal in the morning!

RIPE APPLES: A daily apple can also improve your performance under the sheets, among many other advantages. It's not just that it can keep the doctor away. What is the effect of eating an apple on increasing libido and sex drive? An important factor in increasing sexual stamina and endurance is the high concentration of antioxidants found in apples.

LOBSTERS AND CRABS: Seafood and crustaceans come up again. For their ability to lessen erectile dysfunction, they are well known. They also enhance testosterone production in your body, which increases sex drive and stamina. Libido then rises as a result of this.

RED MEAT: It increases your libido and sex drive and has high zinc content. Over all other meats, including poultry and fish (which is high in important minerals), red meat is generally thought to be healthier.

STRAWBERRIES: Strawberries are a romantic favorite, especially when they're covered in whipped cream or dipped in chocolate. Because of their high vitamin C content, they may increase libido, improve blood flow, and reduce tension and anxiety. Additionally, it facilitates the release of more oxytocin, which is linked to sexual arousal and orgasm and is commonly referred to as the "love" hormone.

CITRUS FRUITS: Oranges and lemons come to mind. Numerous vitamins and minerals can be found abundantly in them. Vitamin C, which is necessary for causing your body's blood flow to accelerate, is something they consistently give you.

MACA: The maca plant, which is native to the Peruvian highlands, has been used for centuries to increase fertility. According to current research, its root may enhance sexual desire. The plant's phytonutrients may improve sexual function and sperm count. Powdered maca root is a popular product. It tastes earthy and nutty. It goes well with yogurt, salads, soups, baked goods, and smoothies.

THE IDEAL SEXUAL SWING FOR COUPLES

One partner can be suspended in the air during sex with a sex swing, a kind of harness that lifts and suspends off the floor. According to the description, "It provides excitement and novelty to sex and lovemaking, where you can experiment with new positions and just enjoy the thrill of doing it in a harness rather than the bed."

Let's start with an obvious fact: Having sex swings is a lot of fun. Right there! We stated as much! We'll admit that not every sexual experience is the same, even though there are many options available and they're all enjoyable in different ways. Certain are superior to others. We therefore have some incredible options for you to check at if you're searching for the best sex swing.

WHAT THINGS SHOULD YOU CONSIDER BEFORE PURCHASING A SEX SWING?

The ideal style for you will depend on your needs and your willingness to splurge. There are many various styles to pick from. For example, single hook swings are available that, well, attach to the ceiling with a single hook. These are excellent for precisely positioning and whirling your partner. Double hook swings are a good option, though, if you'd like a little more stability. A door swing would be a better choice if you don't like the sound of drilling holes in your ceiling and attaching hardware to it. When the door is closed, these bad boys, who go over the top of the door, will hold it in place. As an alternative, you can simply purchase regular slings that are fastened to a strong metal frame. Although these may be more substantial, you won't have to worry about breaking any parts of your house.

The amount of support the sex swing will offer, the amount of space you have in your house, the weight limit, and, of course, the cost are other factors to take into account. Before making your purchase, all of these factors need to be taken into account. Although it's simple to get carried away by the moment, you should use reason and common sense when making this purchase. You will get a sex swing that fits you and not just the first one that catches your eye if you keep these things in the back of your mind. One of the best ways to liven up your sex life is to try this.

TOP SELECTIONS FOR SEXUAL SWINGS

The Strict Leather Premium Sex Sling + Chain Kit from SexSwing.com is an excellent place to start if you'd like to stick with a straightforward and approachable sex swing. It is essentially a cozy-looking seat with swing-back and swing-forward chains attached to the side. Sounds like a typical playground swing, right? That is, sort of, almost. Granted, you'll never have more grown-up fun on a playground than you will on THIS swing. For extra naughty fun, you can even use it to restrain your partner's wrists and ankles. Comparably, the Purple Reins Sex Sling puts comfort first so that you can feel safe and supported while getting sexy. It allows for tight restraint around the wrists and ankles and holds you like a hammock. It may not be the greatest for experimenting with different positions, but it's ideal for beginners who want to feel safe.

You should consider the Fetish Fantasy Spinning Sex Swing if you'd like to try something a little more understated. You get a few straps that support the weight of whoever is inside in place of a seat. This facilitates easy access to all areas of your partner's body. If it doesn't appear sturdy, don't worry—it won't let you down. Even with a spring included, this single hook swing gives you a little bounce when you spin. Ideal for any position you decide on.

The Sportsheets Door Sex Swing Kit is the ideal option if space is limited but you still want to experiment and liven things up. That brings us to our final point. As long as the door is closed, the clips on this one that cross the top of your door will keep it securely in place. Although it appears flimsy and strappy, that is part of its appeal. With this slender and sensual swing, you'll feel especially bound and constrained. Even better, your bank account will be happy as well as you will find it to be among the best deals around. Many people have expressed satisfaction with these swings, each of which is amazing in its own right. In addition to them, repeatedly. There are a plethora of other options available; we have just mentioned a handful. Finding the ideal sex swing for you and your partner truly comes down to exploring and experimenting. We can almost assure you that purchasing them will not be regret because they are a fun addition to the bedroom.

IN CONCLUSION

You're already headed in the right direction if you're thinking about ways to appease your partner. Making an effort to find more engaging ways for your partner to have sex can help prevent your relationship from fizzling out. Assess your sexual preferences and be open with your partner about it. Try new things and pay attention to your partner's sexual arousal when they share it with you. You can improve the quality of your marriage and please your spouse sexually by learning, listening, and growing as a couple.